A PRACTICAL GUIDE
TO CLINICAL SUPERVISION
IN GENETIC COUNSELING

T0177586

Genetic Counseling in Practice

General Editors: Bonnie Jeanne Baty and Angela Trepanier

A Practical Guide to Clinical Supervision in Genetic Counseling

Patricia McCarthy Veach
Distinguished Teaching Professor Emerita
Department of Educational Psychology
University of Minnesota
Minneapolis, MN, USA

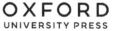

Oxford University Press is a department of the University of Oxford. It furthers
the University's objective of excellence in research, scholarship, and education
by publishing worldwide. Oxford is a registered trade mark of Oxford University
Press in the UK and certain other countries.

Published in the United States of America by Oxford University Press
198 Madison Avenue, New York, NY 10016, United States of America.

Library of Congress Cataloging-in-Publication Data
Names: Veach, Patricia McCarthy, author.
Title: A practical guide to clinical supervision in genetic counseling /
Patricia McCarthy Veach.
Other titles: Genetic counseling in practice.
Description: New York, NY : Oxford University Press, [2023] |
Series: Genetic counseling in practice |
Includes bibliographical references and index.
Identifiers: LCCN 2022034961 (print) | LCCN 2022034962 (ebook) |
ISBN 9780197635438 (paperback) | ISBN 9780197635452 (epub) |
ISBN 9780197635469 (online)
Subjects: MESH: Genetic Counseling—organization & administration |
Personnel Management—standards | Staff Development—standards |
Administrative Personnel—standards | Administrative Personnel—ethics
Classification: LCC RB155.7 (print) | LCC RB155.7 (ebook) | NLM QZ 52 |
DDC 362.196/042—dc23/eng/20220902
LC record available at https://lccn.loc.gov/2022034961
LC ebook record available at https://lccn.loc.gov/2022034962

DOI: 10.1093/med/9780197635438.001.0001

9 8 7 6 5 4 3 2 1

Printed by Marquis, Canada

Contents

Preface

Genetic counseling supervision is central to student professional development, and it is a prevalent activity among genetic counselors. Genetic counselors without question are experts at providing genetic counseling services. A good practitioner, however, is not automatically a good supervisor. Although there are many parallels between genetic counseling practice and supervision, they are not the same activities. Genetic counseling literature supports formal training for supervisors to increase their confidence and maximize their supervision skills. Furthermore, the Accreditation Council for Genetic Counseling (ACGC; 2019a), which endorses genetic counseling graduate programs in North America, requires programs to prepare students to "understand the methods, roles and responsibilities of the process of clinical supervision of trainees" (p. 7).

This book is intended to serve as a practical resource to inform educational efforts and to promote individual supervisors' professional development. Each chapter offers specific suggestions and experiential activities for strengthening and maintaining competencies that promote effective supervision processes and outcomes. The content is pertinent for individual readers and for workshop and classroom instruction. The Appendix, "Instructional Tips for Building Supervision Training Opportunities," contains general suggestions to facilitate the learning experiences of current and future genetic counseling supervisors.

There are four important considerations. First, the book emphasizes student supervision, but basic concepts and skills are relevant for individuals providing supervision to all types of supervisees. Second, the content is applicable for individuals at varying levels of supervision experience—students, novice and experienced supervisors, and individuals interested in becoming supervisors. Third, readers will see the terms "client" and "patient" throughout the chapters. "Client" is consistent with revisions to the ACGC standards and Practice-Based Competencies. This term reflects the variety of settings in which genetic counseling practice and supervision occur. "Patient" is consistent with terminology used in cited publications. Fourth, it is possible that some readers will expect supervisors to masterfully utilize every approach described in this book. Perfectionistic expectations not only cause undue stress but also impede supervision processes and outcomes.

This book is informed by firsthand experiences conducting clinical supervision trainings and providing supervision, as well as existing literature on clinical supervision. Several individuals merit particular recognition: Carrie Atzinger, Ian M. MacFarlane, Krista Redlinger-Grosse, and Katie Wusik shared their expertise by serving as authors for three chapters. Carrie also provided valuable editorial suggestions for other chapters. Nancy Callanan, Bonnie LeRoy, and Casey Reiser (advisors to the book) and Bonnie Baty and Angie Trepanier (genetic counseling series co-editors) are deeply experienced genetic counselors, supervisors, educators, and researchers who reviewed chapter drafts and provided insightful suggestions that enhanced the final product. Finally, I thank the supervisors, practitioners, and students I have had the privilege to work with throughout the years; their perspectives have greatly enriched my understanding of clinical supervision.

Patricia McCarthy Veach, PhD, LP

About the Authors

Carrie Atzinger, MS, CGC, LGC, is an associate professor and co-director of the University of Cincinnati Genetic Counseling Graduate Program (GCGP). She has co-authored 15 peer-reviewed articles, the majority of which are related to topics of supervision in the genetic counseling field or development of genetic counseling self-efficacy. In addition to her teaching, research, and administrative roles in the Cincinnati GCGP, she has co-led workshops in supervision at national meetings and outside universities and hospitals.

Ian M. MacFarlane, PhD, LP, is a licensed psychologist and Research Assistant Professor at the University of Minnesota. He is Director of Admissions and Associate Director of Research for the Genetic Counseling Training Program, member of the Genetic Counseling Workforce Working Group Task Force on Supervision Training, and a founding member of the Advisory Board for the international Clinical Supervision Research Collaborative. His teaching and research include supervision, training, clinical competency, and professional development of genetic counselors and other human services professionals. He has authored 31 professional articles and a genetic counseling research book and has conducted supervisor trainings at 13 genetic counseling programs.

Patricia McCarthy Veach, PhD, LP, is a licensed psychologist and Emerita Professor at the University of Minnesota. She is a member of the Academy of Distinguished Teachers at the University of Minnesota and recipient of the Minnesota Psychological Association Outstanding Graduate Faculty in Psychology Award. Her teaching and research involve supervision, training, and professional development of genetic counselors and other human services professionals. She has authored three books and more than 150 professional articles, taught a graduate-level course on clinical supervision for 30 years, and conducted more than 90 trainings on supervision.

Krista Redlinger-Grosse, PhD, LP, LGC, is a licensed genetic counselor and psychologist who is on faculty with the University of Minnesota Genetic Counseling Training Program as the Director of Fieldwork and Supervisory Training. She also works as a psychologist in private practice providing long-term support to individuals and families impacted by genetic conditions. Her interests center around the integration of the fields of genetic counseling and psychology through clinical work, education, supervision training, and research. She conducts regular workshops to support supervisory development on topics that include feedback and evaluation, boundaries, communication, and cultural engagement.

Katie Wusik, MS, CGC, LGC, is a licensed genetic counselor at Cincinnati Children's Hospital Medical Center. In the past, she has served as the Clinical Coordinator for the University of Cincinnati Genetic Counseling Program. She continues to supervise genetic counseling students in direct and nondirect patient care rotations. Her research focuses on genetic counseling supervision and genetic counselor professional development.

Contributors

Carrie Atzinger, MS, CGC
Co-Director and Associate Professor
Division of Human Genetics/Department of Pediatrics
Cincinnati Children's Hospital Medical Center/University
of Cincinnati College of Medicine
Cincinnati, OH, USA

Ian M. MacFarlane, PhD, LP
Research Assistant Professor
Genetics, Cell Biology and Development
University of Minnesota
Minneapolis, MN, USA

Patricia McCarthy Veach, PhD, LP
Distinguished Teaching Professor Emerita
Department of Educational Psychology
University of Minnesota
Minneapolis, MN, USA

Krista Redlinger-Grosse, PhD, LP, LGC
Director of Fieldwork and Supervisory Training, Genetic
    Counseling Training Program
Department of Genetics, Cell Biology, and Development,
    Institute of Human Genetics
University of Minnesota
Minneapolis, MN, USA

Katie Wusik, MS
Genetic Counselor
Division of Human Genetics
Cincinnati Children's Hospital Medical Center
Cincinnati, OH, USA

Introduction to Supervision Theory and Practice

PATRICIA MCCARTHY VEACH

Objectives

- Define supervision and its functions.
- Present the Reciprocal-Engagement Model of Supervision (REM-S).
- Describe empirically derived genetic counseling supervisor competencies.
- Explain the importance of genetic counselors taking on the role of supervising students.

What Is Clinical Supervision?

When you hear the term *supervision*, what comes to mind? Maybe you think of words such as guidance, support, advice, teaching, consultation, feedback, and evaluation. Supervision can be any of these things in different situations with different supervisees. As such, supervision is a complex activity requiring deliberate self-reflective practice. Furthermore, although there is a certain amount of overlap, the skills of effective supervision are distinct from the skills of genetic counseling practice.

Clinical supervision is the lynchpin of student preparation in human services professions. Many descriptions of this essential activity exist—for example:

[Supervision is] a highly significant activity of mentoring, guiding, and shaping the next generation of competent [genetic counselors].

—GRANT ET AL. (2012, P. 539)

Clinical supervision is an intervention provided by a more senior member of a profession to a more junior colleague or colleagues who typically (but not always) are members of the same profession. This relationship is evaluative and hierarchical, extends over time, and has the simultaneous purposes of enhancing the professional functioning of the more junior person(s); monitoring the quality of professional services offered to the clients, that she, he, or they see; and serving as a gatekeeper for the particular profession the supervisee seeks to enter.

—BERNARD AND GOODYEAR (2014, P. 9)

Clinical supervision is an essential component of genetic counseling education, serving three primary purposes: (1) promoting the professional development of student supervisees who are the genetic counselors of the future, (2) ensuring continued provision of quality professional services, and (3) serving a gate keeper function regarding those individuals who enter the profession.

—MCCARTHY VEACH AND LEROY (2009, P. 401)

Clinical supervision serves to teach, through reflective practice, how to convey genetic information in an understandable, informative and sensitive manner so patients can make informed decisions about genetic testing and management for their conditions.

—WHERLEY ET AL. (2015, P. 702)

These descriptions characterize clinical supervision functions and processes as

- a means of transmitting skills, knowledge, and attitudes of a particular profession through a *focus on behavior* (Bernard & Goodyear, 2014; Grant et al., 2012; Wherley et al., 2015);
- a *relationship* in which one person's skills/professional identity are enhanced by interaction with another (Grant et al., 2012);
- an ongoing *process* in which one experienced person helps another person acquire and maintain appropriate professional/work behavior (Weil, 2000);
- an essential way of ensuring clients receive a *standard of care* (Bernard & Goodyear, 2014; McCarthy Veach & LeRoy, 2009); and
- an activity that fosters professional development across an individual's career (see "Peer Group Supervision" in Chapter 15).

Who Does Supervision Serve?

Supervision serves several constituents (McCarthy Veach & LeRoy, 2009): students, the students' current and future genetic counseling clients, genetic counseling training programs, the genetic counseling profession, and supervisors. The needs of these various constituents require supervisors to wear several "hats" (Bernard & Goodyear, 2014): Supervisors are *skill builders*, helping students develop and maintain skills required of entry-level genetic counselors. They are *socializers*, helping students learn and adopt values, attitudes, and behaviors consistent with the genetic counseling profession. Supervisors are *monitors* of services provided by students to ensure a standard of care for clients and other consumers of genetic counseling services. They are *gatekeepers*, contributing to decisions about who has the necessary characteristics and skills to enter the profession.

A colleague of mine has said, "Genetic counseling is easy, it's genetic counseling student supervision that's challenging." Why is that? I think it is partly because of those multiple hats. Every action we engage in as supervisors should be to serve the needs of our constituents, but sometimes those needs compete. I recommend you inform students at the beginning of your relationship about the nature of the various hats you wear (see the discussion of information agreements in Chapter 3). Furthermore, to minimize misunderstandings, it sometimes helps to tell a student when you are switching hats. For example:

> *Scenario*: The supervisor and student agreed the student would present testing options to the client, but during that part of the counseling session, the supervisor stepped in. Later, when debriefing the session, the student brought up the step-in.
>
> *Student*: You told the client about whole exome sequencing, and I was just getting to that.
>
> *Supervisor*: I know you were well-prepared to present all of the options, and you're disappointed about not getting to do that. Because we were running short on time, I put on my "client care" hat and stepped in. Presenting information within a set time frame is challenging. In retrospect, what do you think you might have done differently to present options more concisely?
>
> [Student offers some ideas, and the supervisor reinforces feasible ones and adds their own thoughts.]
>
> *Supervisor*: Why don't we role play the part of the session where you presented options, so you can try out some of these ideas.

In this example, the supervisor acknowledges the student's disappointment/frustration, clarifies the step-in was not because the student was unprepared, and identifies time management as the reason for the step-in. They go on to normalize the challenging nature of time management, elicit the student's thoughts about how to do things differently, and suggest a practice opportunity. Of note, it is generally a good idea to discuss "step-ins" during debriefings because students may have very different ideas about why you stepped in and what it "says" about their performance.

Reciprocal Engagement Model of Supervision

If I have a [model], I will have a method. I will know what to look for, what to do, and when to do it. I will be able to justify my intervention.

—JANSON (1998, P. 46)

A model of supervision practice provides a conceptual framework for "initiation of the supervision relationship, identification of goals and tasks, and evaluation of supervision processes and outcomes . . . [and] can promote consistency in student training and evaluation within and across genetic counseling programs" (Wherley et al., 2015, p. 703). A model of supervision creates a framework for a seemingly overwhelming endeavor (Kennedy, 2000a). A model also contributes to the "safety net" valued by genetic counseling students to ensure quality client care while allowing students to develop new skills (Hendrickson et al., 2002).

In 2007, McCarthy Veach et al. published an empirically derived Reciprocal-Engagement Model (REM) of clinical genetic counseling practice (shown in Figure 1.1). They based the model on a consensus meeting of genetic counseling program directors or their representatives, key informants, and a review of literature. The REM consists of three key components, five tenets (fundamental assumptions or beliefs), 17 goals specific to genetic counseling sessions, and three broad outcomes.

In 2015, Wherley et al. proposed the Reciprocal-Engagement Model of Supervision (REM-S) to provide a framework for supervising genetic counseling students. Based on the belief that

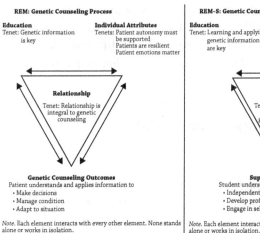

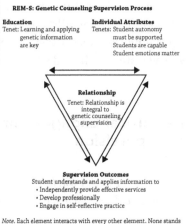

REM: Genetic Counseling Process

Education
Tenet: Genetic information is key

Individual Attributes
Tenets: Patient autonomy must be supported
Patients are resilient
Patient emotions matter

Relationship
Tenet: Relationship is integral to genetic counseling

Genetic Counseling Outcomes
Patient understands and applies information to
• Make decisions
• Manage condition
• Adapt to situation

Note. Each element interacts with every other element. None stands alone or works in isolation.

REM-S: Genetic Counseling Supervision Process

Education
Tenet: Learning and applying genetic information are key

Individual Attributes
Tenets: Student autonomy must be supported
Students are capable
Student emotions matter

Relationship
Tenet: Relationship is integral to genetic counseling supervision

Supervision Outcomes
Student understands and applies information to
• Independently provide effective services
• Develop professionally
• Engage in self-reflective practice

Note. Each element interacts with every other element. None stands alone or works in isolation.

FIGURE 1.1

Comparison of the Reciprocal-Engagement Model of genetic counseling practice (McCarthy Veach et al., 2007) and the Reciprocal-Engagement Model of Supervision.

Source: Wherley, C., McCarthy Veach, P., Martyr, M., & LeRoy, B. S. (2015). Form follows function: A model for clinical supervision practice in genetic counseling. *Journal of Genetic Counseling, 24,* 702–716 (Figure 1, p. 704). Reprinted with permission from the *Journal of Genetic Counseling.*

"form follows function," the REM-S is interconnected with and complementary to the REM of genetic counseling practice. The REM-S helps supervisors "deliberately direct genetic counseling through supervision by structuring supervision to reflect the intended structure of counseling and/or by modeling desired behaviors in interactions with supervisees" (Wherley et al., 2015, p. 703). The supervision structure allows supervisors to teach, model, and reinforce each REM element.

Three REM-S components align with those of the REM (see Figure 1.1): "(1) education to guide student skill development and ensure they provide a standard of patient care, (2) relationship development, and (3) individual student attributes. Each focus is equally important and interacts with the others" (Wherley et al., 2015, p. 704). These components are realized through five tenets and 16 associated goals. The goals are informed by genetic counseling supervisor competencies (Eubanks Higgins et al., 2013), described later in this chapter, as well as by literature in medicine and psychology. Three broad outcome goals involve the student being able to understand and apply information to (1) independently provide effective services, (2) develop professionally, and (3) engage in self-reflective practice.

REM-S Tenets and Goals

Tenet 1: Learning and applying genetic information are key. Important activities include building and refining students' case assessment skills, psychosocial skills, and teaching skills. There are three goals: (1) supervisor knows what information to impart, (2) supervisor teaches genetic counseling knowledge and skills, and (3) student acquires and/or draws upon knowledge and skills to provide genetic counseling services appropriately.

Tenet 2: Relationship is integral to genetic counseling supervision. Supervision is a relationally based process. Good communication is essential to the process, and the supervisor is a positive part of the process. There are three goals: (1) supervisor and student establish a bond, (2) good supervisor–student communication occurs, and (3) supervisor and student characteristics positively influence the supervision process.

Tenet 3: Student autonomy must be supported. This tenet assumes students know themselves best and should be active participants to the extent possible in exercising choice. Also, the supervisor respects and values each student within their personal, professional, and cultural contexts. There are four goals: (1) establishment of a supervision agreement/ contract; (2) integrate personal, professional, and cultural context into the supervision relationship and decisions;

(3) student feels empowered and more in control; and (4) facilitate collaborative decisions.

Tenet 4: Students are capable. This tenet reflects a belief that the vast majority of students possess the abilities and qualities necessary to become competent genetic counselors. They have the capacity to learn and grow from supervised clinical experiences tailored to their developmental level. There are three goals: (1) recognize student stage of development, (2) tailor supervision to student skill level, and (3) foster student confidence.

Tenet 5: Student emotions make a difference. Students have emotional reactions to the challenges of learning in supervision and in response to patients' emotions. The supervisor (and student) must attend to the emotional impact of the supervision process. It is also critically important for supervisors and students to connect in a human way. There are three goals: (1) supervisor and student know student concerns, (2) both supervisor and student understand supervisor–student and student–patient dynamics, and (3) supervisor addresses student's feelings and responses to supervision and genetic counseling.

REM-S Supervisor Strategies

In a study of practicing genetic counselor supervisors, Suguitan et al. (2019) identified 14 strategy domains (broad topic areas) that align with REM-S tenets and goals. The strategy domains are shown in Box 1.1.

The three most prevalent strategy domains across the REM-S goals were assessment of student, practice self-reflection to increase supervisor self-awareness, and establish student goals and expectations. Table 1.1 contains a list of the most prevalent strategy domains for each REM-S goal and examples of individual strategies. Suguitan et al. (2019) concluded that due to the reciprocal nature of the REM-S, any given strategy may help achieve multiple goals. Furthermore, skill practice opportunities combined with feedback are overarching strategies to help students achieve learning goals.

BOX 1.1 Genetic Counselor Strategy Domains That Align with REM-S Tenets and Goals

Assessment of student

Assist students in collaborating with other health professionals

Empower student

Establish student goals and expectations

Establish good communication with student

Establish working alliance with student

Facilitate patient care with student

Gather information from/with student

Give information to student

Practice self-reflection to increase supervisor self-awareness

Provide culturally competent supervision

Provide pre- and post-clinical sessions

Provide resources to student

Use psychosocial counseling skills/strategies in supervision

Source: Suguitan, M. D., Redlinger-Grosse, K., McCarthy Veach, P., & LeRoy, B. S. (2019). Genetic counseling supervisor strategies: An elaboration of the Reciprocal-Engagement Model of Supervision. *Journal of Genetic Counseling, 28*, 602–615.

Supervisor Competencies

Eubanks Higgins et al. (2013) conducted a modified Delphi study to establish basic competencies (knowledge, skills, and qualities) for genetic counseling clinical supervisors. Program directors and assistant directors of accredited genetic counseling programs in North America and clinical supervisors rated the importance of competencies derived from supervision literature in allied health professions. Participants rated 142 competencies as important for supervisors. The researchers classified these competencies within

TABLE 1.1 Summary of the Most Prevalent Strategy Domains and Examples of Specific Strategies Organized by REM-S Tenets and Goals

REM-S Tenets and Goals	Strategy Domain	Specific Strategy Example
Tenet 1: Learning and applying genetic information is key		
Goal 1: Supervisor knows what information to impart	Practice self-reflection to increase supervisor self-awareness	Give feedback based on patient needs
	Assess student	Assess student development based on previous student rotation performance
	Establish student goals and expectations	Establish goals for session based on student feedback
Goal 2: Supervisor teaches knowledge and skills	Assess student	Assess student performance of specific GC skill
	Facilitate patient care with student	Model GC skills during session
	Empower student	Assign exercises to build confidence
	Give information to student	Provide possible patient perception to student
	Practice self-reflection to increase supervisor self-awareness	Gauge student knowledge and experience levels

TABLE 1.1 (Continued)

REM-S Tenets and Goals	Strategy Domain	Specific Strategy Example
Goal 3: Student acquires skills and/or draws upon knowledge appropriately	Assess student	Evaluate student knowledge from activity
	Provide pre- and post-clinical sessions	Assign self-reflection activity post-clinic
	Practice self-reflection to increase supervisor self-awareness	Use self-awareness on supervisor emotions
Tenet 2: Relationship is integral to genetic counseling supervision		
Goal 1: Supervisor and student establish a bond	Establish student goals and expectations	Establish student goals for the rotation
	Gather information from/with student	Ask question about student's perceived strengths
	Collaborate with health professionals	Introduce student to professional health team
	Establish good communication with student	Discuss communication styles with student
Goal 2: Good supervisor–student communication	Establish good communication with student	Facilitate bi-directional communication with student
	Collaborate with health professionals with student	Facilitate student evaluation with other supervisors
	Establish working alliance with student	Establish expectations to increase openness and approachability

(continued)

TABLE 1.1 (Continued)

REM-S Tenets and Goals	Strategy Domain	Specific Strategy Example
Goal 3: Supervisor and student characteristics positively influence process	Provide culturally competent supervision	Build rapport based on shared culture
	Give information to student	Share known patient background to student
	Use psychosocial counseling skills/ strategies in supervision	Use primary empathy (affect)
Tenet 3: Student autonomy must be supported		
Goal 1: Establish supervision agreement/ contract	Establish student goals and expectations	Establish pre-session expectations
	Assess student	Assess student skills based on previous rotation
	Practice self-reflection to increase supervisor self-awareness	Use self-awareness of own genetic counseling style
Goal 2: Integrate personal, professional, and cultural context into the supervision relationship and decisions	Provide culturally competent supervision	Establish session expectations based on cultural context
	Give information to student	Provide anticipatory guidance on how culture informs decision-making
	Use psychosocial counseling skills/ strategies in supervision	Use self-disclosing statement (e.g., I would do it this way)

TABLE 1.1 (Continued)

REM-S Tenets and Goals	Strategy Domain	Specific Strategy Example
Goal 3: Student feels empowered and more in control	Empower student	Use positive reinforcement
	Use psychosocial counseling skills/ strategies in supervision	Address student defense mechanisms
	Facilitate patient care with student	Intervene in student-led session based on student reaction
Goal 4: Facilitate collaborative decisions	Establish student goals and expectations	Establish patient follow-up with student
	Gather information from/with student	Check-in with student post-session
	Assess student	Compare assessments between other supervisors
	Practice self-reflection to increase supervisor self-awareness	Draw insights from previous supervision experiences
Tenet 4: Students are capable		
Goal 1: Recognize student stage of development	Practice self-reflection to increase supervisor self-awareness	Use self-reflection about student readiness
	Assess student	Quiz student knowledge
	Gather information from/with student	Ask questions about student self-assessment

(continued)

TABLE 1.1 (Continued)

REM-S Tenets and Goals	Strategy Domain	Specific Strategy Example
Goal 2: Tailor supervision to student skill level	Practice self-reflection to increase supervisor self-awareness	Reference personal experience as a student
	Assess student	Evaluate student's case preparation
	Gather information from/with student	Assess quality of case preparation/outline
Goal 3: Foster student confidence	Empower student	Respect student's autonomy in session
	Use psychosocial counseling skills/ strategies in supervision	Use advanced empathy
	Facilitate patient care with student	Intervene in student-led session upon student request
Tenet 5: Student emotions make a difference		
Goal 1: Supervisor and student know student concerns	Use psychosocial counseling skills/ strategies in supervision	Ask questions about student concerns
	Practice self-reflection to increase supervisor self-awareness	Recognize supervisor–student boundaries
	Establish good communication with student	Discuss student reaction post-session

TABLE 1.1 (Continued)

REM-S Tenets and Goals	Strategy Domain	Specific Strategy Example
Goal 2: Both supervisor and student understand supervisor–student and student–patient dynamics	Establish good communication with student	Discuss communication preferences with student
	Collaborate with health professionals with student	Utilize program director
	Establish working alliance with student	Establish clinic expectations with student and other supervisors
Goal 3: Supervisor addresses student's feelings and responses to supervision and genetic counseling	Use psychosocial counseling skills/ strategies in supervision	Use primary empathy (content)
	Practice self-reflection to increase supervisor self-awareness	Recognize limits of one's supervisory role
	Establish good communication with student	Discuss countertransference post-sessions

Note: Every REM goal had at least three prevalent strategies. For some REM goals, there were ties for the third most prevalent domain; in those cases, four or five strategy domains are listed.

GC, genetic counseling.

Source: Suguitan, M. D., Redlinger-Grosse, K., McCarthy Veach, P., & LeRoy, B. S. (2019). Genetic counseling supervisor strategies: An elaboration of the Reciprocal-Engagement Model of Supervision. *Journal of Genetic Counseling*, *28*, 602–615 (Table 4, pp. 611–612). Reprinted with permission from the *Journal of Genetic Counseling*.

six domains (broad topic areas) and 15 categories (more specific topics within domains):

Domain 1: Personal Traits and Characteristics. Domain 1 consists of 23 competencies reflecting supervisor general qualities and behaviors such as possessing demonstrated knowledge of the genetic counseling practice-based competencies (Accreditation Council for Genetic Counseling [ACGC], 2019a), showing commitment to supervising, seeking training opportunities in supervision methods, and engaging in lifelong learning and professional development.

Domain 2: Relationship Building and Maintenance. Domain 2 reflects supervisor "qualities and behaviors that promote a working alliance and a safe and positive learning environment" (Eubanks Higgins et al., 2013, p. 44). There are 29 competencies across four categories: *facilitative characteristics* (e.g., empathy, genuineness, and respect), *initiation of the supervisory relationship* (e.g., orienting students to supervision and clarifying supervisor expectations), *supervision dynamics* (are sensitive to the evaluative nature of supervision and inherent power differential, and expect, recognize, and address student anxiety), and *conflict resolution* (e.g., recognize and address disagreements that inevitably arise).

Domain 3: Student Evaluation. Domain 3 includes 26 competencies within four categories reflecting supervisor effective engagement in *goal setting* (e.g., setting realistic learning goals through discussion with students, and identifying student learning needs), *evaluation* (e.g., specifying and explaining evaluation criteria, and using evaluation tools effectively), *feedback* (e.g., providing timely, specific, honest feedback and helping students process feedback), and *remediation* (e.g., recognizing and documenting problematic performance as needed, and interacting with program faculty to discuss difficulties with students).

Domain 4: Student Centered Supervision. Domain 4 involves the supervisor working effectively with student characteristics such as learning style, developmental level, and cultural background. There are 32 competencies divided into two categories: *use of appropriate methods and techniques* (e.g., providing a balance of challenge and support appropriate to a student's developmental level and experience, and using supervisory methods appropriate to a student's level of conceptual development) and *facilitation of student development* (e.g., encouraging students to develop their own personal genetic counseling styles, and encouraging multicultural readings and educational opportunities).

Domain 5: Guidance and Monitoring of Patient Care. Domain 5 consists of competencies for fostering student learning about how to provide a standard of care. There are 20 competencies across three categories: *documentation* (e.g., provides guidance to students about effectively documenting clinical encounters, and stresses the importance of accurate and timely medical documentation), *case preparation* (e.g., assists students in developing a counseling plan and prioritizing goals in the plan, and assists students in incorporating patient psychological and behavioral characteristics into the genetic counseling session), and *counseling interventions and post-counseling debriefing* (e.g., assists students in adjusting counseling goals for a patient based on ongoing assessment and evaluation during the genetic counseling session, and elicits students' perceptions of patient psychosocial dynamics).

Domain 6: Ethical and Legal Aspects of Supervision. Domain 6 involves the supervisor modeling ethical and professional treatment of patients and students. There are 12 competencies across two categories: *professional conduct* (e.g., demonstrates ethical and professional standards of genetic counseling practice, and seeks appropriate consultation in ethically ambiguous situations) and *nature and boundaries of supervision* (e.g., communicates knowledge of ethical considerations pertinent to supervision relationships, and maintains confidentiality with those outside the site about student evaluation and feedback).

Appendix 1A contains the individual competencies within each domain and category.

Supervision Is Hierarchical

Both the REM-S (Wherley et al., 2015) and Eubanks Higgins et al.'s (2013) supervisor competencies reflect the hierarchical nature of the supervisor–student relationship. Within this hierarchy, supervisors are in the more powerful seat because they are the genetic counseling experts and ultimate evaluators of student performance and readiness to move forward. As supervisors, we should be ever mindful of the power differential when approaching supervision and use this power in intentional ways. One way to be intentional is to think about how you develop working relationships with the individuals for whom you provide genetic counseling services and consider ways you might apply those behaviors with students:

- Cultivate an attitude of respect, openness, and sensitivity to build and maintain a positive working alliance. A strong working alliance has been shown to be related to stronger supervisee self-efficacy regarding their genetic counseling skills (Caldwell et al., 2018b).
- Expect that students are there for the "right" reasons, namely learning and developing professionally.
- Believe in students' ability and resilience. Most will have the necessary capacity to become genetic counselors and will be able to withstand the challenges that come with learning and refining their skills.

- Recognize that supervision is a very emotional process. Both your students and you will experience anticipation, hope, anxiety, frustration, and joy at various times throughout your relationship.
- Deliver "difficult news" (corrective feedback) with honesty, clarity, and compassion.

Why Serve as a Supervisor?

The National Society of Genetic Counselors' (NSGC, 2018) Code of Ethics and the ACGC's (2019a) practice-based competencies "either explicitly state or imply genetic counselors have a duty to supervise or work with genetic counseling students" (Reiser, 2019, p. 727). These documents reflect that "only genetic counselors can impart to students the art and skill of genetic counseling" (Reiser, 2019, p. 728).

Supervision is an essential training component of the genetic counseling profession, and it is a prevalent activity among genetic counselor practitioners. In 2021, the NSGC's Professional Status Survey found that 40% of 3,006 respondents provided supervision to students. Moreover, student supervision was among the top three significant roles of those in direct patient care positions.

Although there are potential challenges to supervision (e.g., it takes time and effort, and some genetic counselors may believe they are too busy with other tasks) (Berg et al., 2018; Reiser, 2019), research supports numerous benefits from serving as a supervisor (Berg et al., 2018). Benefits include playing a role in shaping the profession's evolution, reduced client caseload, increased confidence about one's genetic counseling skills (Hendrickson et al., 2002), and the enjoyment of teaching and contributing to the profession (Lindh et al., 2003). Serving as a supervisor helps "keep you on your toes" (Lindh et al., 2003), promotes your own professional development, and promotes the vitality of the field by helping prepare future generations of genetic counselors. Supervision may also help offset professional risks such as compassion fatigue because it provides a break from challenging clinical work (Udipi et al., 2008). Additional potential benefits include accruing professional activity credits for recertification and recognition by some institutions through the awarding of faculty status (Reiser et al., 2019).

Closing Thoughts

As this chapter suggests, much is expected of genetic counseling supervisors. The following chapters contain practical suggestions for strengthening and maintaining competencies that promote effective supervision processes and outcomes.

Learning Activities

Most learning activities can be adapted for dyad or small group discussions or for written exercises. Time estimates are provided for discussions, but additional time should be allotted for large group processing.

Activity 1.1 Supervisor Self-Assessment

The Psychotherapy Supervisor Development Scale (PSDS; Watkins et al., 1995) provides a baseline of where you presently see yourself with respect to your supervision competency/effectiveness and supervisor identity/commitment or where you anticipate you will be when you begin serving as a supervisor.

Complete the PSDS and use the Scoring Key contained in Appendix 1B. Then share your responses with a partner.

Estimated time: 15 minutes

Note: Novices can retake this scale after undergoing further supervision training/experience to gauge their development. Experienced supervisors can note specific items for which they feel less effective/committed and set goals to increase their effectiveness/commitment.

Activity 1.2 Reflecting on Supervision

Take turns discussing these questions with a partner:

- What are three feelings you have about being (becoming) a supervisor?
  - If you are currently a supervisor, how, if at all, have your feelings changed over time?
- What do you think are the two most important qualities of a supervisor? Why?
- What do you think are the two most important qualities of a supervisee? Why?
- What are two personal qualities you think stand out/will stand out about you as a supervisor?
- What are/will be two of your biggest growth edges as a supervisor?
- What is/will be your biggest challenge as a supervisor?

Estimated time: 20 minutes

Note: This activity can be followed by a whole group discussion. If doing a whole group discussion, do not require participants to share their responses to the questions about personal qualities and growth edges.

Activity 1.3 Wearing Different Supervisor Hats

For each of the following scenarios, (1) identify which supervisor hat you would put on to address the situation and (2) write down what you would say. Write your response as if you are speaking directly to the individual in the scenario. Share your responses with a partner or in small groups.

- The student you are supervising in a rotation has midterms next week and is behind on case preps for the upcoming clients.
- Your student shows up for their first day in clinic in blue jeans and flip-flops and says they didn't have time to do their laundry. Your clinic has a dress code policy that the student had received previously.
- A student you supervised in their final rotation asks you to serve as a reference for various jobs to which they have applied and says they hope you will give them a strong endorsement. Your evaluation of their performance during the rotation was mixed.
- The student you are supervising has come to clinic 10 minutes late multiple times stating difficulty in getting up in the morning because of not being able to sleep at night. This student also revealed they have an ongoing struggle with depression.
- During a counseling session, you realize your student did not update a counseling plan and agenda as you instructed when you reviewed this with them earlier in the week. You needed to step in to provide more relevant and correct information to the client about testing options.
- The program director of the training program your student is in reaches out to get your feedback on the student's psychosocial skills.

Estimated time: 30 minutes

Note: These scenarios can also be used as role plays.

Activity 1.4 Genetic Counseling Supervisor Competencies

For each domain, describe two specific behaviors you do/could do as a supervisor to demonstrate some aspect of the competency. Discuss your responses with a partner.

Domain 1: Personal Traits and Characteristics—Supervisor is a competent genetic counselor, as evidenced by their training, education, and certification. Supervisor demonstrates a variety of personal qualities and related skills.
1.
2.

Domain 2: Relationship Building and Maintenance—Supervisor demonstrates knowledge and skills that promote a working alliance and a safe and positive environment.
1.
2.

Domain 3: Student Evaluation—Supervisor demonstrates knowledge and skills that reflect awareness of and effective management of the evaluative nature of supervision.
1.
2.

Domain 4: Student Centered Supervision—Supervisor demonstrates knowledge and skills that allow them to work effectively with students' individual differences, in particular, student learning styles and developmental levels.
1.
2.

Domain 5: Guidance and Monitoring of Patient Care—Supervisor demonstrates knowledge and skills in ensuring students learn to provide a standard of patient care.
1.
2.

Domain 6: Ethical and Legal Aspects of Supervision—Supervisor demonstrates knowledge and skills that model ethical and professional treatment of patients and students.

1.

2.

Estimated time: 40 minutes

Source: Eubanks Higgins, S., McCarthy Veach, P., MacFarlane, I. M., Borders, L. D., LeRoy, B. S., & Callanan, N. (2013). Genetic counseling supervisor competencies: Results of a Delphi study. *Journal of Genetic Counseling, 22*, 39–57.

Activity 1.5 REM-S Goals

Review the individual REM-S goals listed in Table 1.1.

- List three supervision goals that are most comfortable for you (i.e., goals you believe you are/will be able to achieve fairly often).
- Next list three supervision goals with which you are least comfortable (i.e., goals you believe are/will be challenging for you to achieve).
- Review the goals with which you are least comfortable. Do they have anything in common? What makes them challenging for you?
- Identify one or two things you could do to increase your comfort with each challenging goal.
- Discuss your responses with a partner.

Estimated time: 40 minutes

Appendix 1A
Genetic Counseling Supervisor Competencies

Genetic counselor supervisors strive to facilitate the development of competent entry-level genetic counselors through supervised clinical experiences. Genetic counselor supervisors demonstrate knowledge and skills commensurate with the American Board of Genetic Counseling (ABGC, 2004) practice-based competencies, which include communication, critical thinking, interpersonal, counseling, psychosocial assessment skills, and professional ethics and values. In addition, the following are characteristics, knowledge and skills of effective supervisors of students in genetic counseling.

I. Personal Traits and Characteristics

Genetic counselor supervisors are competent genetic counselors as evidenced by their training, education and certification. They demonstrate a variety of personal qualities and related skills.

Genetic Counselor Supervisors

- Demonstrate knowledge and skills commensurate with the ABGC practice-based competencies
- Recognize that care of the patients is their primary responsibility
- Are highly competent, ethical in practice and supervision, accessible to students, comfortable in the authority inherent in the supervisory role, flexible, transparent, and patient
- Have problem-solving abilities and a sense of humor
- Demonstrate a commitment and desire to supervise and seek opportunities for training in supervision techniques and methods

- Advocate for students in the clinical setting
- Model appropriate professional behavior through appropriate dress and demeanor
- Demonstrate effective time management in practice and supervision
- Demonstrate knowledge of individual differences with respect to gender, race, ethnicity, culture, sexual orientation, spirituality or religion, and age, and understand the importance of these characteristics in supervisory relationships
- Explore their own cultural identity and how this identity affects their values and beliefs about counseling and supervision
- Have knowledge about the particular genetic counseling program for which they are supervising students, including the overall objectives, evaluation process, and the supervisor's role
- Keep up to date with changes in practice, new genetic technologies, and trends in the profession
- Maintain a commitment to lifelong learning and professional development, including knowing their strengths and weaknesses as a genetic counselor and supervisor

II. Relationship Building and Maintenance

Genetic counselor supervisors demonstrate knowledge and skills that promote a working alliance and a safe and positive learning environment.

Facilitative Characteristics

Genetic Counselor Supervisors

- Are encouraging, motivating, and respectful
- Are empathic, genuine, concrete, and immediate (give swift attention to feedback and other student issues)

Initiation of the Supervisory Relationship

Genetic Counselor Supervisors

- State the purpose of supervision
- Conduct an orientation which includes either a verbal or written contract with students regarding the details of the clinical placement and supervisory relationship
- Describe their supervisory style to students and provide them with information about their own credentials
- Delineate supervisor expectations and explain when and how supervision will occur
- Clarify roles of genetic counselors at the site in the supervision process
- Explain the roles of other professionals (e.g., counselors, psychologist, physicians, social workers)
- Engage with students to establish a mutually trusting relationship/working alliance

Supervision Dynamics

Genetic Counselor Supervisors

- Recognize that some student anxiety is normal and seek to lessen students' anxieties and help students find productive ways to manage anxiety
- Recognize and address transference and countertransference issues in supervision in ways that are productive for the supervision process
- Recognize that student resistance is a normal response to challenge, growth, and change and deal with resistance in productive ways
- Are sensitive to the evaluative nature of supervision and the power differential inherent in the process and effectively respond to students' anxieties regarding performance evaluations

- As needed, explore the student's tendencies to over-identify with a patient or supervisor
- Elicit and are open to candid and ongoing feedback from the student about the supervision experience

Conflict Resolution

Genetic Counselor Supervisors

- Recognize that some level of disagreement is inevitable in supervisory relationships and use key principles of conflict resolution to attend to conflicts that interfere with the supervision process
- Resolve problems with interpersonal dynamics that arise by creating an action plan (to include contact with genetic counseling program faculty as needed)
- Provide students with information about due process when they disagree about feedback or a rotation evaluation (e.g., check with other genetic counseling supervisors on site, talk with genetic counseling program faculty, etc.)

III. Student Evaluation

Genetic counselor supervisors demonstrate knowledge and skills that reflect awareness of and effective management of the evaluative nature of supervision.

Goal Setting

Genetic Counselor Supervisors

- Recognize that planning and goal setting are critical components of the supervisory process
- Set realistic learning goals through discussion with students
- Identify learning needs of students at various levels of training and experience

- Use the ABGC practice-based competencies in setting goals
- Initiate a renegotiation of rotation goals if needed
- Incorporate into goals:
  - The student's self-identified areas of weakness
  - The student's past clinical experiences
  - The student's report of feedback from previous supervisors
  - The student's developmental level
  - The student's learning priorities
  - Opportunities available at the particular site

Evaluation

Genetic Counselor Supervisors

- Specify and explain criteria used to determine if a student meets expectations set by the site and/or genetic counseling program
- Engage in active listening and observing during sessions
- Identify student's areas of strengths and weaknesses
- Evaluate student performance and skill development for purposes of grade assignment or completion of a rotation
- Use evaluation tools to effectively document student skill development and progress during the course of a rotation
- Evaluate interpersonal dynamics among genetic counseling staff, other clinical and non-clinical personnel, patients, and students
- Collaborate with other genetic counseling colleagues also supervising the student if compiling a mid-point or final evaluation
- Provide a summative evaluation as a progress report to students midway through rotation
- Provide a final summative evaluation which includes topics discussed in previous evaluations

Feedback

Genetic Counselor Supervisors

- Elicit students' thoughts and feelings regarding clinical skills and respond in a manner that enhances the supervision process
- Provide both verbal and nonverbal supportive feedback
- Strive to provide to students in a timely manner and private area, feedback that is clear, specific, honest, and objective
- Provide feedback about student behavior rather than personal traits the student cannot change
- Prioritize feedback based on student developmental level
- Comment on positive changes made by students in response to feedback
- Help students process both immediate and summative feedback

Remediation

Genetic Counselor Supervisors

- Recognize student impairment and take steps to document if needed
- Interact with genetic counseling program faculty to discuss difficulties with students
- As needed, collaborate with genetic counseling program faculty to create for students with impairment, interventions relevant to areas of deficit
- As needed, provide information about consequences of underperformance

IV. Student Centered Supervision

Genetic counselor supervisors demonstrate knowledge and skills that allow them to work effectively with student individual differences, in particular, student learning styles and developmental levels.

Use of Appropriate Methods and Techniques

Genetic Counselor Supervisors

- Provide a balance of challenge and support appropriate to student developmental level and experience
- Adjust rotation activities such as conferences, projects or other assignments based on the student's learning needs, training, experience, area of interest, and conceptual development
- Use supervisory methods appropriate to student's level of conceptual development, training and experience
- Ensure that students have an appropriate amount and type of clinical duties
- Encourage student autonomy, as appropriate
- Expect students to own consequences of their actions with patients and supervisors
- Assign students to patient referrals or roles in sessions that are appropriate to the student's developmental level and experience
- Make a plan with the student for progression from observation to participation in genetic counseling sessions
- Model effective collaboration and communication skills in an interdisciplinary team
- Understand the value of providing students with multiple observation opportunities and allow students to observe whether they are in a beginning or advanced rotation
- Engage in varied supervisory interventions (e.g., role playing, role reversal, live supervision, modeling, brain-storming, advising, reporting on cases)
- Take on various supervisory roles as needed (e.g., teacher, counselor, consultant, advisor, mentor, coordinator, evaluator)
- Create learning opportunities in subject matter that is lacking during the course of the rotation

- Demonstrate ability to communicate critical reasoning behind clinical practice decisions
- Effectively co-counsel with students
- Effectively evaluate and share knowledge with students in the form of new educational materials, literature, and patient educational materials
- Elicit new alternatives from students for solutions, techniques and responses to patients

Facilitation of Student Development

Genetic Counselor Supervisors

- Encourage development of critical reasoning skills
- Understand the developmental nature of supervision
- Promote student self-evaluation, self-exploration, and problem-solving abilities
- Encourage students to develop their own personal styles of genetic counseling
- Help students develop teamwork skills
- Discuss with students current professional issues in genetic counseling
- Incorporate individual student learning styles and feedback preferences into the supervision process
- Conduct self-assessment after sessions as a means of modeling professional growth for the student
- Encourage multicultural readings and educational opportunities

V. Guidance and Monitoring of Patient Care

Genetic counselor supervisors demonstrate knowledge and skills in ensuring students learn to provide a standard of patient care.

Documentation

Genetic Counselor Supervisors

- Provide guidance to students in effectively documenting clinical encounters
- Emphasize the importance of accurate and timely medical documentation
- Provide guidance to students in identifying appropriate information to be included in a verbal or written report
- Provide guidance to students in adapting verbal and written reports for the work environment and type of communication (to patient, to physician, etc.)

Case Preparation

Genetic Counselor Supervisors

- Guide students in case preparation
- Assist students in developing a counseling plan and prioritizing goals in the plan for patients
- Assist students in obtaining and appropriately reviewing medical records, patient education materials and testing information
- Require students to consider relevant ethical issues and cultural considerations in planning for sessions
- Facilitate students' understanding of when and how to work with an interpreter for linguistically diverse patients
- Facilitate the discussion and use of current research in patient care
- Facilitate understanding of the difference between clinical and research-based genetic testing and implications for patients
- Assist students in incorporating patient psychological and behavioral characteristics into the genetic counseling session

Counseling Interventions and Post-Counseling Debriefing

Genetic Counselor Supervisors

- Intervene during sessions to direct students towards presenting information in a logical, concise, and clear manner as needed to ensure patient care
- Assist students in adjusting counseling goals for a patient based on ongoing assessment and evaluation during the genetic counseling session
- Assist students in determining whether the objectives for the patient have been met
- Guide and evaluate students' abilities to permit the patient to express intense emotional states and help students manage extreme patient behaviors
- Elicit students' perceptions of patient psychosocial dynamics
- Help students process and learn effective coping strategies for emotionally difficult cases

VI. Ethical and Legal Aspects of Supervision

Genetic counselor supervisors demonstrate knowledge and skills that model ethical and professional treatment of patients and students.

Professional Conduct

Genetic Counselor Supervisors

- Are ethical in practice and supervision
- Demonstrate ethical and professional standards of genetic counseling practice (e.g., confidentiality, duty to warn)
- Seek appropriate consultation in situations of ethical uncertainty

- Demonstrate knowledge of the professional Code of Ethics of relevant professional organizations such as the National Society of Genetic Counselors (NSGC) and Canadian Association of Genetic Counsellors (CAGC)
- Communicate an understanding of legal and regulatory documents and their impact on the profession (e.g., HIPPA, informed consent)

Nature and Boundaries of Supervision

Genetic Counselor Supervisors

- Communicate knowledge of ethical considerations that pertain to the supervisory relationship (e.g., multiple role relationships, due process, confidentiality)
- Clearly define the boundaries of the supervisory relationship
- Avoid simultaneous roles in addition to supervision with students (i.e., teacher, research mentor, employer, friend) or monitor them for negative effects on students when unavoidable
- Maintain confidentiality from those outside the site about student evaluation and feedback
- Explain the rationale and/or boundaries around addressing the student's personal issues during the supervision process

Source: Eubanks Higgins, S., McCarthy Veach, P., MacFarlane, I. M., Borders, L. D., LeRoy, B. S., & Callanan, N. (2013). Genetic counseling supervisor competencies: Results of a Delphi study. *Journal of Genetic Counseling, 22*, 39–57. Reprinted with permission from the *Journal of Genetic Counseling.*

Appendix 1B
The Psychotherapy Supervisor
Development Scale

Please respond to each of the following items by circling the number that best reflects your current view of yourself as a supervisor. There are no right or wrong answers. If you have not yet served as a supervisor, anticipate how you would view your competency and identity.

	Never		Half the time			Always
	1	2	3	4	5	6	7

1. I consider the supervision relationship that I provide to be helpful to my supervisees.   1 2 3 4 5 6 7

2. Becoming and being a supervisor demands a commitment (i.e., to keep working at developing oneself as supervisor) that I believe I have made.   1 2 3 4 5 6 7

3. I have a realistic awareness about my strengths and abilities as a supervisor.   1 2 3 4 5 6 7

4. Sometimes I believe I'm just playing at being a supervisor.   1 2 3 4 5 6 7

5. When needed, I am able to be appropriately assertive and confrontive with my supervisees.   1 2 3 4 5 6 7

6. I just don't consider myself that identified with the supervisor role.   1 2 3 4 5 6 7

7. I believe I am able to increasingly foster a sense of self-sufficiency in my supervisees.   1 2 3 4 5 6 7

8. Becoming a supervisor is an ongoing process that requires much time and energy, but I see myself as well on my way to getting there.   1 2 3 4 5 6 7

9. Right now I feel ill-at-ease and somewhat confused with the supervisor role.   1 2 3 4 5 6 7

10. I believe I have a good knowledge of and understanding about the supervision process itself.   1 2 3 4 5 6 7

11. I consider supervision to be a very important role that I perform.   1 2 3 4 5 6 7

12. I believe I have a good awareness about myself as a supervisor, the impact that I have on supervisees, and how I affect the supervisory situation as a whole.   1 2 3 4 5 6 7

13. I believe I am generally effective in dealing with transference/countertransference issues in supervision.   1 2 3 4 5 6 7

14. If asked, "Do you really feel like a supervisor?", I could honestly answer "Yes."   1 2 3 4 5 6 7

15. I have a realistic awareness about my strengths and abilities as a supervisor.   1 2 3 4 5 6 7

16. As a supervisor, I structure
    the supervision experience
    effectively.   1   2   3   4   5   6   7

17. If asked, "Can you give a good
    assessment of yourself as a
    supervisor?", I could easily
    answer "Yes."   1   2   3   4   5   6   7

18. I must say that, when I
    perform my supervisory
    responsibilities, I often
    think of myself as an imposter. 1   2   3   4   5   6   7

The Psychotherapy Supervisor Development Scale

Scoring Instructions

To determine your score, sum up the numbers that you circled for each item.

Please note that Items 4, 6, 9, and 18 should be reverse scored.

Scores can range from 18 to 126, with higher scores indicating greater development defined as competency/effectiveness and identity/commitment.

Note: Revised "counseling/psychotherapy supervisor" to "supervisor." *Source*: Watkins, C. E., Jr., Schneider, L. J., Haynes, J., & Nieberding, R. (1995). Measuring psychotherapy supervisor development: An initial effort at scale development and validation. *The Clinical Supervisor*, 13, 77–90. Reprinted with permission from *The Clinical Supervisor*.

2

Supervisory Styles

PATRICIA MCCARTHY VEACH

Objectives

- Describe major supervisory styles.
- Identify support and guidance as dynamics common to all supervisory styles.

If someone asks you what other kind of relationship is most similar to supervision, what type of relationship would you name? Is it one of the relationships shown in Box 2.1, or some other type of relationship?

The relationship you identify says a lot about your attitude and approach to supervision, including your preferred style, perceptions of your responsibilities and the student's responsibilities, and the ways in which power and trust influence your interactions.

Stylistic Differences

Hart and Nance (2003) define *style* as the distinctive way supervisors respond to supervisees and the different approaches they use. People are unique in the ways they think, feel, and act, so it is not surprising that supervisors (and their supervisees) vary in

BOX 2.1 Types of Relationships

Expert–apprentice
Coach–athlete
Rock climber–belayer
Parent–child
Choreographer–dancer
Teacher–student
Director–actor
Conductor–musician
Judge–defendant
Therapist–client

how they approach supervision. Consider the following potential areas of focus in supervision, and ask yourself to what extent you emphasize or think you would stress each one:

- The student's feelings about their clients
- Conceptualizing client needs
- What the student did in sessions and what strategies would have been more effective
- The working relationship between the student and yourself and how that is affecting the student's performance
- Sharing your own developmental process and learning as a genetic counselor

Bernard (1979) describes three distinct styles in her Discrimination Model of supervision: consultant, teacher, and counselor. She broadly defines each style as follows:

The supervisor as consultant focuses on a relationship with the counselor that is explorative in nature and assumes that the counselor has the ability to express his or her supervision needs. The supervisor as teacher focuses on some knowledge or expertise that he or she wishes to transmit to the counselor. The supervisor as counselor places priority on the counselor's personal needs, with the belief that this focus will allow the counselor to overcome the nervousness or self-doubt that impedes natural development. (p. 64)

Other authors have proposed a fourth style—supervisor as evaluator (McCarthy Veach & LeRoy, 2009). Although I recognize, as do others (e.g., Bernard & Goodyear, 2014), that evaluation is always present in supervision, there are times when it is particularly salient. In the next sections, I draw from the work of Bernard (1979, 1997; Bernard & Goodyear, 2014) and McCarthy Veach and LeRoy (2009) to elaborate on the characteristics of different supervisory styles.

Consultation Style

In a consultation style, supervisor and student interactions are *collaborative*. The consultant supervisor is a *facilitator* who engages with the student to determine mutually agreed upon goals, plans, and actions and encourages the student to self-evaluate. Consultation activities include discussing client needs and options for addressing them; brainstorming strategies and interventions; and supervisor self-disclosure of their own learning, mistakes, challenges, and successes. Either the supervisor or the student may "go first" in sharing their ideas. Given the collaborative nature of a consultation style, the supervisor and student share responsibility for determining the agenda and problem-solving, and the balance of power in the relationship is more equal compared to other styles. In most cases, however, students are likely to still perceive a power differential between themselves and their supervisor.

Example

> *Consultee*: I would like to figure out how to respond when clients are angry. I've thought of some things I might try, but I'm not sure they'll work.
>
> *Consultant*: Angry clients are challenging for me, too. I find it's sometimes helpful to acknowledge their feelings with a reflection statement. What sorts of things have you thought about doing?

Teaching Style

In a teaching style, interactions are grounded in *instruction*. The supervisor acts as a *resource*, imparting knowledge and skills and usually takes the lead in establishing the supervision agenda. Teaching activities include modeling, explaining, conceptualizing client needs and identifying appropriate interventions, and providing insights during debriefings. The teacher supervisor is the *expert* and, as such, possesses a great deal of power in the relationship. Novices typically prefer a teaching style because it provides them with a foundation on which to develop their genetic counseling skills (see Chapter 5). Bernard's teaching style implies a *directive teacher* (e.g., demonstrating and explaining).

A directive teacher instructs by leading—that is, offering their perspective first. There is another type of teaching style that I call *evocative teaching*. An evocative teacher leads by following—asking the student to share their perspective first, followed by the supervisor shaping and/or adding to the student's perspective.

Example

> *Student*: Some of my clients call me "honey" and "dear," and when I'm in the middle of explaining something, they'll stop to tell me I'm doing fine. I'm beginning to think they'll never take me seriously.

Directive teacher: Some clients pick up on students' uncertainty. They can tell a lot from nonverbals. For the next client, try sitting in a more relaxed way, look at her when you speak instead of at your notes, and keep your voice calm but firm.

Evocative teacher: What do you suppose they might be picking up on from your nonverbals? [*Student responds.*] How do you think you could modify those behaviors with the next client? [*Student responds.*] Your idea to look at the client more often is a good strategy. I think that may be easier to do if you put your notes aside occasionally during the session.

Time and other considerations sometimes require a "quick" answer, and in those situations, a directive style may be the better approach. Giving a student a critical piece of information, or telling the student where to find that information, provides an expedient solution. An evocative approach promotes deeper learning and self-supervision. By "asking" rather than "telling" whenever feasible, students have an opportunity to practice self-reflection. An evocative style builds student confidence and competencies, encourages independent functioning, and makes the work of supervision a shared endeavor.

Counseling Style

In a counseling style, the supervisor and student interactions involve *exploration*. The supervisor is a *prompter* of self-awareness about personal issues affecting students' work. Counselor supervisors are *not* therapists. They are not responsible for helping students resolve personal issues. Rather, supervisors help students recognize and manage their issues as they affect their professional work. For instance, a student has difficulty with authoritarian figures due to a harsh upbringing. During sessions in which clients bring a family member who is domineering, the student tends to allow that individual to speak for the client. The counselor supervisor would help the student recognize and understand this behavior pattern and discuss how to manage it in the future. The counselor supervisor also encourages students to recognize and navigate common developmental tasks (e.g., fluctuating self-confidence). Counseling activities include exploring feelings and discussing student reactions and defenses and their impact on service provision. This style usually occurs less frequently in genetic counseling supervision.

Example

> Counselee: When the patient started talking about being diagnosed with cancer, all I could think about was how they weren't that much older than me.
>
> Counselor: How were you feeling as you listened to their experience?" [Student responds.] And how did your feelings affect what you said or did next? [Student responds.] What might you do the next time you feel that way with a patient?

Note that in this example, the counselor supervisor's focus is on how the student's feelings impact their behaviors during the session. The discussion of what to do next time similarly focuses on behaviors rather than on addressing the feelings.

Evaluation Style

In an evaluation style, the supervisor–student interactions involve *appraisal*. The supervisor is an *assessor* of the students' work, the genetic counseling services provided, and the supervision relationship. Activities include formal and informal assessment (e.g., mid- and final-rotation evaluations), goal setting, and giving and receiving feedback. The ways these activities happen reflect the other styles (e.g., the supervisor tells the student their impressions [directive teacher], the supervisor begins by asking the student for their impressions [evocative teacher], the supervisor and student mutually determine ratings on an evaluation form [consultant], the supervisor invites the supervisee to share their feelings about the feedback they received [counselor]).

Example

> *Evaluatee*: I gave the couple the referral to a support group, but I don't think they'll follow-through on it. I think I could have done it better.
>
> *Evaluator*: It's great you recognized this. I think you sounded apologetic when you gave the referral, and that may have given an impression that they shouldn't waste their time. A stronger recommendation would increase the chances of follow-through. How could you have said things differently?

Note, in this example, the supervisor affirms the student's attempt to self-evaluate (which helps build self-supervision skills) and reinforces the accuracy of that self-evaluation. These strategies are consistent with an evaluation style. The supervisor goes on to direct the student's attention to a possible reason for an unsuccessful referral and encourages the student to consider an alternative way to present referrals. These strategies are consistent, respectively, with directive teaching and evocative teaching styles. As noted later in this chapter, "mixing styles" commonly occurs in supervision interactions.

Style Limitations

Each supervisory style has potential limitations. A consultation style usually is preferred by more experienced students who have achieved some sense of the genetic counseling work and gained confidence in their ability to offer input in collaborative interactions. Furthermore, if not used strategically, interventions such as supervisor self-disclosure may lack relevance to the goals of supervision and/or shift the focus from the student.

Strategies consistent with a directive teaching style, such as telling or modeling, may indicate *what* to say or do, but they do not always help students learn *why* and *how* to engage in the desired behaviors. Also, when used frequently, directive teaching may lower the student's self-confidence by implying they lack the necessary knowledge or skills and lead to dependency on the supervisor for further answers. A directive approach may result in premature closure, preventing students from trying to figure things out for themselves. A directive teaching style places a great deal of responsibility on supervisors and diminishes the "bi-directional" nature of supervision (Wherley et al., 2015). I like to advise directive supervisors to "stop working so hard" and instead use an evocative style, when feasible, to encourage students to engage in the learning process. An evocative teaching style may take more time in the short term compared to a directive style, however, and it may initially raise student anxiety (e.g., they may think you are looking for a certain answer and will criticize them if they get it wrong).

A counseling style may feel uncomfortable for students if they are unaccustomed to sharing feelings and other types of personal information, are surprised to learn their feelings are a relevant supervision topic, and/or fear being judged. An evaluation style can be challenging for supervisors because they tend to be most uncomfortable with evaluation activities, especially those involving corrective feedback (Bernard & Goodyear, 2014). Moreover, despite their actual intentions, some students may perceive everything supervisors say and do as an evaluation.

Given the benefits and potential limitations of each supervisory style, it is often preferable to use a mix of styles, as elaborated on below. In addition, I strongly encourage you to *explain in advance* what your preferred approach is as a supervisor and why. This may require some self-reflection on your part. Explaining your preferred approach is also important because students have style preferences, and their preferences may not match yours.

Additional Comments About Supervisory Styles

There are a few factors to bear in mind when considering supervisory styles and their effects on supervision processes and outcomes.

Styles overlap. Supervisory styles are not discrete. Supervisors and students will often use a mixture of styles in their conversations.

Styles are equally valuable. One supervisory style is not better than another. Each has a place in supervision relationships.

Versatility is key. Ideally, supervisors (and students) are flexible enough to use each style deliberately, based on clear reasons for doing so (Bernard, 1979). As noted by Hart and Nance (2003),

> A style of supervision may and should change from session to session because of the changing needs of the supervisee and the perception of both supervisor and supervisee of that need. Furthermore, styles of supervision may change within each particular supervision session as multiple needs of supervisees emerge. (p. 156)

Necessity should trump preference. In the absence of training and self-reflection, we tend to choose the most comfortable or familiar style for most of our interactions (Bernard, 1979). Yet, as Bernard notes, supervisors (and students) should use these styles intentionally and not based solely on personal preference.

Styles may be reactive. Either person in the supervision relationship can *pull* for a certain style. For supervisors, it is important to assess the student's style and decide whether to accommodate it or use a different style.

Styles may conflict. Hart and Nance (2003) found psychological counseling supervisors and supervisees had clear preferences for certain styles, but there was little agreement between them about those preferences. They also found both supervisors and supervisees expected certain styles to be prevalent in supervision. Tension may arise when the supervisor prefers and uses one style and the student prefers another style (e.g., a student asks what they should say when a client is afraid to discuss testing options [directive teaching style], and the supervisor responds by asking how the student feels when a client is fearful [counseling style]). Discussion of stylistic differences is important to prevent or reduce conflict.

The timing and choosing of different styles are important. When time dictates a brief conversation, the supervisor should deliberately decide which style(s) is most critical. Consider, for example, the following possible supervisor responses and which one you might be inclined to begin with:

Student: The patient's speech was so slurred from myotonic dystrophy that I had trouble understanding him. I hated to keep asking him to repeat himself. I was half-tempted to just pretend that I understood.

Possible supervisor responses:

Consultant: That's a tough situation. It's so easy to feel anxious, especially since it's obvious how frustrated they are. Why don't we come up with some ideas of how to handle this in the future?

Directive teacher: Next time try addressing it directly with the patient. For example, say something like, "It must be frustrating to have to repeat things for me." Getting the issue out in the open will make you feel less anxious and better able to understand him.

Evocative teacher: What stopped you from pretending you understood? [*Student responds.*] So, you knew pretending would not have worked. Now that you have time to think about it, what might you have done?

Counselor: What were you *saying to* yourself about not understanding this patient? [*Student responds.*] How did that affect the way you felt and what you did?"

Evaluator: Your concern for this patient is a real strength. [Pause] What do you think would have happened if you pretended to understand?

Situations requiring a more in-depth discussion are likely to involve responses reflecting multiple styles. You should consider which style to begin with to set the stage for the subsequent use of other styles. For example, in discussing plans for an upcoming client, you might first elicit student feelings about the client's situation (counselor); then ask what the student thinks about how to best approach the client (evocative teacher); give positive feedback to the student about their conceptualization of the case (evaluator); add your ideas about approaching the client (directive teacher); and, finally, brainstorm a few opening statements for establishing rapport with the client (consultant).

Behaviors Common to Supervisory Styles

Research has identified *support* and *direction* as universal behaviors present in all supervision styles to varying degrees (e.g., Hart & Nance, 2003). Hart and Nance (2003) described support as a focus on *supervisee* concerns about themselves and their feelings and thoughts when working with clients. Support behaviors include empathy and rapport and trust building, among others. These authors described direction as focusing on conceptualizing *clients* and on counseling techniques/interventions. Direction behaviors include, for instance, questions, giving instructions, and challenging the supervisee.

Bernard's teaching, counseling, and consulting styles have been mapped onto continua of support and direction behaviors (e.g., Bernard & Goodyear, 2014; Hart & Nance, 2003). Table 2.1 contains an adaptation of that work to reflect the styles of evocative teacher, directive teacher, consultant, and counselor.

Notice the consultant style is on the lower end of the continua for support and direction. This does not mean the supervisor is uninvolved in the process. Hart and Nance (2003) state,

The supervisor gives low support and low direction, believing that the supervisee already possesses sufficient emotional

TABLE 2.1 Continua of Supervisor Behaviors

	Higher Direction	Lower Direction
Higher Support	Evocative teacher	Counselor
Lower Support	Directive teacher	Consultant

Support: Focuses on *student* concerns about self and feelings and thoughts when working with clients.

Direction: Focuses on conceptualizing *clients* and on counseling techniques.

Adapted from Hart, G., & Nance, D. (2003). Styles of counselor supervision as perceived by supervisors and supervisees. *Counselor Education & Supervision*, 43, 146–158.

awareness of himself or herself and adequate skill in client conceptualization and counseling techniques. The focus is on the supervisee's integration of his or her existing skills with a caring, but not intrusive or directive, manner. (p. 149)

The evaluation style does not fit into just one area of the continuum for either support or direction. As noted previously, the evaluator style overlaps with the other styles with respect to how the supervisor and student approach feedback, goal setting, and evaluation. Therefore, behaviors consistent with evaluation will vary in the amount of support and direction they provide.

Closing Thoughts

Supervision relationships with genetic counseling students usually are brief (a few weeks) and can be intense given the nature of genetic counseling work. As discussed in Chapter 3, students are interested in knowing your supervisory style, and I suggest you reflect upon and inform them about your preferences. I also recommend you try to discern student preferences early on. An obvious strategy is to ask them directly. Students with prior genetic counseling and supervision experience may be able to tell you with some accuracy. Regardless of a student's experience level, another useful strategy is to pay attention to how they engage with you in your initial interactions. Their behaviors will give valuable clues as to their general preferences.

Learning Activities

Most learning activities can be adapted for dyad or small group discussions or for written exercises. Time estimates are provided for discussions, but additional time should be allotted for large group processing.

Activity 2.1 Identifying Supervisory Styles

For the following scenario, identify which supervisory style is most predominant. Next indicate which supervisor response you prefer and explain why. Discuss your responses in small groups. (Appendix 2A lists the predominant style reflected in each response.)

> *Scenario*: During the family history portion of a session that the student was conducting, the client stated their mother had died in a car accident 2 months ago. In response, the student wrote down the information and moved on to the next question on their agenda.
> During debriefing, your student says, "The mother's death wasn't relevant to their reason for seeking genetic counseling. Plus, I wasn't sure what I should say about it."
> *Supervisor*: Perhaps you were uncomfortable addressing their loss? Let's talk about how you were feeling in that moment and how it influenced what you did.

Supervisor: It's important to acknowledge their loss before moving on in the history gathering. I would have said . . .

Supervisor: It seems like your scientist lens told you their mother's death was not relevant to their genetic risk, while your counselor lens told you it's important to acknowledge their loss. Those are great realizations. . . . [Pause] What might you do differently the next time you have two competing thoughts?

Supervisor: I'm happy to share my ideas, but first I'd like to hear your thoughts about what you might have said or done differently.

Supervisor: When patients share stories of trauma and loss, I think of those as my "cue" to stop what I was doing or where I may have been going in the session and address their feelings. Why don't we brainstorm together some ways you could do that.

Estimated time: 20 minutes

Note: Participants can also write their own response if they do not prefer any of the ones listed and identify what style(s) is evident in their response.

Activity 2.2 Using Supervisory Styles

For each of these situations, construct a response to the student that is consistent with each of the supervisor styles. Write your response as if you are speaking directly to the student.

Situation 1: Regarding a pregnant client, the student says, "She looked at me and point blank said, 'How could you possibly understand? I'll bet you don't have any children.' I didn't know what to say."

How might you respond if you wanted to take a(n):
Evocative teacher approach?

Directive teacher approach?

Counselor approach?

Consultant Approach?

Evaluator Approach?

Situation 2: The student says, "Well, I know that the patient's first baby had anencephaly diagnosed by ultrasound. So, when the tech began the ultrasound, she started to cry. I told her not to worry, but I don't think it helped very much."

How might you respond if you wanted to take a(n):

Evocative teacher approach?

Directive teacher approach?

Counselor approach?

Consultant approach

Evaluator approach?

Situation 3: The student says, "The patient's husband stepped in and answered all the questions I had for her. She seemed okay with that, but I think I should have addressed it, only I didn't know how."

How might you respond if you wanted to take a(n):

Evocative teacher approach?

Directive teacher approach?

Counselor approach?

Consultant approach

Evaluator approach?

Situation 4: The student says, "I wanted to engage the patient's partner in the discussion of hereditary cancer testing options, but he was obviously not interested. He just kept reading his newspaper."

How might you respond if you wanted to take a(n):

Evocative teacher approach?

Directive teacher approach?

Counselor approach?

Consultant approach

Evaluator approach?

Situation 5: The student says, "I wasn't ready for how angry the doctor got when I told her testing children for the genetic form of early onset Alzheimer disease wasn't available in our lab."

How might you respond if you wanted to take a(n):

Evocative teacher approach?

Directive teacher approach?

Counselor approach?

Consultant approach

Evaluator approach?

Situation 6: The student says, "I have to admit I had a hard time knowing how to respond when the patient was so upset to learn her daughter has Turner syndrome. It just seems to me that so many of our patients have disorders that are far more serious."

How might you respond if you wanted to take a(n):

Evocative teacher approach?

Directive teacher approach?

Counselor approach?

Consultant approach

Evaluator approach?

Activity 2.3 Supervisory Focus and Style

Think about the way you typically provide supervision (or think you would provide supervision if you have not yet done so) and indicate your level of agreement with each statement. Try not to think about one particular supervisee when you complete this questionnaire. There are no right or wrong answers. Use this scale to respond to each item:

1: Strongly Disagree; 2: Disagree; 3: Agree; 4: Strongly Agree

		SD	D	A	SA
1.	I would refer the supervisee to appropriate readings from counseling texts.	1	2	3	4

2. I would want to establish mutually
determined goals for the content of
each supervisory session. 1 2 3 4

3. I would devote considerable attention
to the supervisee's feelings about
client cases. 1 2 3 4

4. I would answer the supervisee's
questions about client sessions as
directly and clearly as possible. 1 2 3 4

5. I would give the supervisee examples
of possible ways to handle client
concerns. 1 2 3 4

6. I would focus on the counselor's
interpersonal dynamics as illustrated
in relationships with clients. 1 2 3 4

7. I would remain flexible during
supervision to give advice and direct
feedback or to explore personal issues. 1 2 3 4

8. I would suggest we role-play counseling
interactions that the supervisee has
described. 1 2 3 4

9. I would use empathy as an important
supervisory tool. 1 2 3 4

10. I would brainstorm with the supervisee
possible conceptualizations of clients'
concerns. 1 2 3 4

11. I would encourage the supervisee to ask
questions about whatever information
I conveyed during the supervision
session. 1 2 3 4

12. I would direct attention to the
supervisee's relationship with me and
would try to draw parallels between our
relationship and the counselor–client
relationship. 1 2 3 4

13. I would encourage the supervisee to speak about their past history and learning experiences.   1   2   3   4

14. I would treat supervision relatively informally, much like a discussion between two colleagues.   1   2   3   4

15. I would give examples from both readings and from my own experience to illustrate the points I wish the supervisee to remember.   1   2   3   4

16. I would review counseling sessions and offer my reactions and feedback.   1   2   3   4

17. I would be certain to mention at least several reactions/ideas/suggestions regarding what might be done in future counseling sessions.   1   2   3   4

18. I would behave in much the same manner with the supervisee as I behave with most of my clients.   1   2   3   4

19. I would use self-disclosure of my own client cases and my own personal emotional reactions with clients.   1   2   3   4

20. I would attempt to aid the supervisee to feel more adequate during future counseling sessions.   1   2   3   4

21. I would allow the supervisee to reject or accept my feedback; the supervisee would be allowed to choose how/if my ideas might be implemented with clients.   1   2   3   4

Use the answer key in Appendix 2A to tally your responses. Then discuss with a partner:

- Do your scores suggest you have a preferred style? If so, which style? Was this what you expected? Why or why not?

- Are your scores across the styles fairly equal? What do you think this says about your approach to supervision?
- Do you have low scores for one or more styles? Why do you think that is? What do you think the implications might be of a low score?
- Does your preferred style(s) as a supervisor bear any relationship to your preferred style as a supervisee?

Estimated time: 30 minutes

Adapted with permission from Yager, G. G., Wilson, F. R., Brewer, D., & Kinnetz, P. (1989). *The development and validation of an instrument to measure counseling supervisor focus and style.* Paper presented at the annual meeting of the American Education Research Association, San Francisco. Unpublished instrument.

Activity 2.4 Supervision Metaphors

Take turns discussing these questions with a partner or in small groups:

- What type of relationship do you think is most similar to supervision? (Refer to Box 2.1 for ideas.)
- How is that relationship similar to supervision? Different?
- Where does the relationship you identified fit on the support and guidance continua shown in Table 2.1?

Estimated time: 15 minutes

Adapted from Fall, M., & Sutton, J. M., Jr. (2004). *Clinical supervision: A handbook for practitioners.* Pearson.

Activity 2.5 The Counselor Supervisory Style

Supervisor instructions: Without giving any information that might identify the student or client(s), briefly describe a supervision situation in which you used a counselor style of supervision with a student. What was the situation? What did the student say? Do? What did you say? Do?

If you are new to supervision, an option is to provide an example from when you were a student.

Student instructions: Without giving any information that might identify the supervisor or client(s), briefly describe a supervision situation in which the supervisor used a counselor style of supervision with you. What was the situation? What did you say? Do? What did the supervisor say? Do?

Note: This exercise can be modified or expanded to include other supervisory styles.

Activity 2.6 Supervisory Styles: Triad Role Plays

Take turns as supervisor, student, and observer for the following scenarios. The supervisor should use one of these styles: evocative teacher, counselor, or consultant. The supervisor should try to use the selected style for most of the role play. After each role play, the student and observer should indicate which style they thought was predominant and provide examples of dialogue consistent with that style.

> *Scenario 1*: You are debriefing a prenatal session in which the student shared with the couple that the child they are expecting has trisomy 18. The couple was visibly upset, and the student became teary-eyed and lost their train of thought. You stepped in to continue the session. During the debriefing, you wish to discuss your step-in with the student.

Scenario 2: You are debriefing a prenatal session in which the student was only able to get one- or two-word answers from the father during the family history taking, and he seemed to become increasingly agitated as the session progressed. The couple agreed to have an amnio, and the student began discussing termination as one option if the results of the amnio are abnormal. The father angrily said, "I told you when we first came in here that we wouldn't consider an abortion under any circumstances. But you went ahead and brought that up anyway!" The student apologized and finished the rest of the session. You could tell, however, that the student was shaken by the father's anger.

Scenario 3: You are debriefing a standardized client session. The client was a 30-year-old woman whose father was recently diagnosed with spinocerebellar ataxia. The student explained there is a test that could reveal whether she also carries the gene mutation for this condition. She responded, "I just couldn't handle hearing that I have it, too. I'll take my chances. My husband and I are trying to have a baby, and I want to concentrate on that. Do you think I'm doing the right thing?" The student told the woman that yes, she was doing the right thing. During the debriefing, the student says the client's question threw them off, and all they could think to say was the first thing that came to their mind.

Note: The person in the supervisor role can choose which style to use (you may wish to encourage them to either use the style with which they are least comfortable or choose the style that seems most appropriate given the scenario), or individuals can be assigned a style.

Estimated time: 30 minutes

Appendix 2A
Learning Activities Answer Key

Activity 2.1 Identifying Supervisory Styles

Response 1: Counselor
Response 2: Directive teacher
Response 3: Evaluator
Response 4: Evocative teacher
Response 5: Consultant

Activity 2.3 Supervisor Focus and Style Inventory Scoring Key

Scoring Key: In each column, sum your responses for these items.

Teaching	Counseling	Consultation
1	3	2
5	6	4
8	9	7
11	12	10
15	13	14
16	18	19
17	20	21
Total:		

Scores for each style can range from 7 to 28. Higher scores indicate a stronger preference for a style.

3

Setting the Stage for Supervision

PATRICIA MCCARTHY VEACH

Objectives

- Discuss the importance of the working alliance and ways to begin establishing a strong working relationship.
- Identify anticipatory guidance strategies to structure supervision.
- Explain the purposes and use of supervision information statements and agreements.

Initiating the Supervisory Relationship

Good supervision is [all] about the relationship.

—ELLIS (2010, P. 106)

Building a Supervision Working Alliance

The supervision relationship is the key conduit to all genetic counseling supervision processes and outcomes (Wherley et al., 2015). *Working alliance*, or working relationship, consists of three elements: agreement on goals, agreement on tasks necessary to complete those goals, and a bond (caring, trust, and rapport) between the supervisor and the supervisee. A stronger bond develops when students perceive the supervisor as caring as much about them as they do about clients and when students believe they can freely share their thoughts and feelings with the supervisor (Shulman, 2006). The working alliance "fosters the training of the supervisee, utilizing the developed skills and knowledge of the supervisor" (Caldwell et al., 2018b, p. 1507). A working alliance begins to form at the very first contact between a supervisor and a student and continues to develop throughout their supervision relationship (Shulman, 2006).

A strong working alliance "is vital to the student's progress in a clinical rotation" (Wherley et al., 2015, p. 708). Caldwell et al. (2018b) surveyed second-year genetic counseling students to examine whether their perceived working alliance was related to their counseling self-efficacy. They found a higher working alliance was significantly related to greater self-efficacy overall, with a stronger connection between these variables for students who had a single supervisor during a rotation. They concluded that supervisors should try to build strong relationships with students to positively influence their self-efficacy about their clinical skills. When a student has more than one supervisor for a setting, it can be helpful for all supervisors to discuss and agree on their expectations.

Supervisor consistency, transparency, and maintenance of professional boundaries build and strengthen the supervisor–student bond, and goal setting promotes agreement on the tasks and outcomes of the student's genetic counseling work and work in supervision. The working alliance is also strengthened when supervisors are genuine, honest, and present with the person they are supervising. Additional supervisor factors affecting the quality of the working alliance include, among others, supervisor style and sources of their interpersonal influence (how expert, trustworthy, and likeable/warm they are perceived to be) (Bernard & Goodyear, 2014; Ellis, 2010; Falender et al., 2014) and their degree of authority (Shulman, 2006). Supervisee factors include, among others, attachment style and emotional intelligence, history of positive and negative supervision experiences, stress level and anxiety, coping resources (Bernard & Goodyear, 2014), and age and experience (Shulman, 2006). Personal traits and cultural background of both supervisors and students are critical factors (see Chapter 4). Good communication between the supervisor and the student is an essential interpersonal ingredient in the development of a strong working alliance (Wherley et al., 2015).

Eubanks Higgins et al. (2013) identified seven supervisor competencies specific to initiating the supervision relationship (see also Chapter 1, Appendix 1A). Supervisors should (1) state the purpose of supervision, (2) conduct an orientation that includes either a verbal or a written contract with students regarding the details of the fieldwork placement and supervisory relationship, (3) describe their supervisory style to students and provide them with information about their own credentials, (4) delineate their expectations and explain when and how supervision will occur, (5) clarify the roles of genetic counselors at the site, (6) explain the roles of other professionals (e.g., counselors, psychologists, physicians, and social workers), and (7) engage with students to establish a mutually trusting relationship/working alliance. These seven competencies are key to creating an initial frame for the supervision relationship.

Prepping for Supervision: Anticipatory Guidance Strategies

When beginning a supervision relationship, what sorts of things do you think help supervisors and students get started? Several initial activities impact subsequent supervision processes and outcomes. Bernard (2010) refers to these activities as *infrastructure*, or "all those matters that, when attended to properly, allow the road of supervision to be clear by lifting any fog caused by disorganization or a lack of important information or a comprehensive supervision plan" (p. 239). Activities that organize the supervision experience "can be as specific as finding time in one's schedule to conduct uninterrupted supervision sessions or as sweeping as establishing performance criteria for the supervisee that will guide the experience" (p. 239).

The extent to which supervisors attend to infrastructure and the ways they do so influence how students anticipate and evaluate the working alliance. Consider the following analogies expressed by student supervisees:

> Being in supervision is like . . .
>
> . . . *hiking up a mountain where at first [supervision] looks daunting, but we are able to pace ourselves and follow those who have tread the path before us, and use leadership and orientation of our leader, the supervisor. We are sure that the view from the top will be wonderful.*
>
> . . . *scuba diving for the first time and not knowing how to run the air tank, so I feel like I am suffocating.*
>
> . . . *being a bug under a microscope.*
>
> . . . *getting onto a rollercoaster—it seems calm at first, but you know that there will be some crazy drops and speeds up ahead.*
>
> . . . *planting a garden—you think you know what you're going to get, but sometimes you are surprised.*
>
> . . . *living in a snow globe that some kid recently shook up—I look forward to all of the snow settling peacefully again.*
>
> . . . *going from the minors to the majors.*

Student and Supervisor Questions

One strategy for beginning to establish a frame for supervision is to consider the kinds of questions students may have about supervision. Student questions are like a "projective test," suggesting what is uppermost in their minds, their feelings about supervision, their priorities, and their uncertainties. Awareness of these questions allows supervisors to anticipate and begin addressing student needs and concerns from the outset. Appendix 3A contains examples of student questions identified by students and supervisors who have participated in supervision trainings. These questions broadly reflect student interest in/uncertainty about the supervisor and the supervisor–student relationship; what the supervisor knows about the student; supervisor background/credentials, personal traits, interpersonal qualities, and supervisory style; supervision processes and methods; supervision logistics and resources; and supervisor expectations about student performance (both the tasks performed and at what skill level).

Supervisors also have questions about their students before beginning a supervision relationship. Supervisors who reflect on their questions are better able to be strategic in structuring the supervision relationship. Appendix 3B contains examples of supervisor questions. These questions indicate supervisor priorities and concerns, interest in the student as a person, and attentiveness to student needs and expectations.

Two overarching "meta-questions" embody students' questions: (1) Will you help me be skilled enough by the end of the rotation? and (2) Will you do anything to hurt me? Two meta-questions encompass supervisors' questions: (1) Are you skilled enough/will you be skilled enough by the end of the rotation? and (2) Will you say or do anything to harm my clients? These questions suggest two critical supervision dynamics—trust and hope. Effective supervision relationships begin with each party believing in the ability and motivations of the other individual and having confidence in the likelihood of a successful outcome.

One way to start addressing student and supervisor questions is through a pre-rotation getting-acquainted activity. You could email five questions to your student and ask them to send you their responses and invite your student to send five questions they would like you to answer. Alternatively, as time permits, you could discuss select questions at your first in-person meeting.

Written information in the form of a statement or an agreement is another strategy for addressing student questions about their supervision experience and for articulating your priorities and concerns.

Supervision Information Statements and Agreements

Supervision information statements and agreements are written documents that can promote the supervision relationship by providing an overview of the supervision experience (McCarthy Veach & LeRoy, 2009) and clarifying expectations (Ellis et al., 2013; Siskind & Atzinger, 2019). A written document serves several functions (McCarthy Veach & LeRoy, 2009): It provides a frame for a highly complex activity; educates students about the nature of supervision; clarifies infrastructure, processes, and desired outcomes; stimulates student questions; promotes common understanding; facilitates supervision processes and outcomes; and formalizes the supervision relationship. Importantly, it sets a "tone" for the evolving supervision relationship. A written document allows you to "front-load" many critical elements of supervision.

In some cases, you may structure this information as a formal supervisor agreement that both you and the student sign. A formal agreement has the added benefit of providing informed consent for supervision because it includes expectations regarding student and supervisor ethical and professional behavior (see Chapter 11). Furthermore, when structured as a signed agreement, it provides a formal record, documenting that the elements were covered with the student.

A written document is a stimulus for an initial meeting with a student and an excellent resource when students have a pressing question and cannot recall the answer (e.g., whom to contact if they are ill and cannot attend clinic). Both information statements and agreements ensure certain key elements are highlighted for every student, and they spare the supervisor having to repeat the same information with each new supervisee. A document can be specific to an individual supervisor. Alternatively, it can be a "group document," created and used by supervisors at a single clinic, except for elements unique to each supervisor (e.g., background and credentials, and supervisor style).

Although written documents cover key elements of supervision, each has a unique "flavor" with respect to which elements are emphasized and how content is expressed. For instance, they can be worded formally and written in the third person (the supervisor, the student), or they can be more informal and written in the first and second person (I, you). The content and wording give students an initial impression of who the supervisor is, what they care about, and what supervision may be like.

Information statements and agreements *are not meant to replace a conversation(s)* between the supervisor and the student. Rather, they help structure initial conversations about expectations and processes. They also are not intended to contain every possible piece of information a student might need. Rather, they include some of the more important types of information. I recommend a document be no longer than two pages of single-spaced text. Table 3.1 outlines typical content areas for written statements and agreements.

Appendix 3C contains an example of an information statement, and Appendix 3D contains an example of a supervision agreement.

Additional Strategies to Set the Stage for Supervision

Several additional strategies may help provide structure, clarity, and preparation for supervision.

Provide observation opportunities. Ask students to observe a counseling session once or twice at your clinic (if allowed) before beginning the rotation.

Assess student preparation. Prepare a pre-rotation quiz or role play to assess knowledge you expect students to know prior to beginning.

Provide guidance on case preps. Give students examples of your case preparations. You could expand on this strategy by having students review the examples and then asking them to share their impressions of content (nature, scope, and amount of detail).

TABLE 3.1 Content Areas for Supervision Information Statements and Agreements

Elements	Topics
Title	May be formal (e.g., "Clinical Supervision Agreement," "Clinical Supervision Statement") or informal (e.g., "Welcome to Supervision")
Professional disclosure	Supervisor credentials or qualifications
Practical issues and logistics	Frequency, length, location, missed supervision time, how to contact you in emergencies, your co-counseling style
Supervision process	Methods and format—when and how you provide feedback; objectives—the types of skills emphasized; roles and responsibilities of each party
Potential benefits and risks	Possible benefits and risks of the supervision process; outcomes the student may experience because of supervision processes
Evaluation/due process	Description of evaluation procedures; due process procedures—to whom can students direct any concerns
Ethical and legal issues	Confidentiality limits; multiple role conflicts; guidelines for client treatment; client charting and follow-up letters
Addendum	Additional statements that arise from supervisor/student discussion of the statement
Statement of agreement	Form is signed and dated by both parties
Typical attachments	Forms used to evaluate the student; professional code of ethics; other forms specific to rotation site

Alternatively, you could have students prep for a case that you also prepare and then compare your notes. You could also ask students to identify portions of the prep they feel more and less comfortable developing for clients. These activities are useful for inviting conversation about differences between "academic" descriptions of case preps and actual case preps for your client population.

Share client letters. Give students examples of client letters. The same expansion described in the "provide guidance on case preps" strategy is applicable for client letters.

Provide written resources. Give students relevant clinic policies (e.g., dress code, transportation and parking information, client bill of rights, documentation rules for students, and schedule expectations). Some policies can be quite technical and "dense." You may wish to highlight the most relevant portions for students. One way to do this is to ask students who are finishing a rotation to identify the portions of the policies they regard as most relevant.

Schedule supervision time in advance. Set dates and times for supervision and make this protected time unless there is a major emergency. Speaking about supervision in social work, Moncho (2013) notes,

> the "high volume, high intensity" [means] supervision is either sacrificed, or done exclusively on the fly. And while supervision on the fly—as supervisor and supervisee pass each other in the hall, run into each other at the coffee machine, or otherwise track each other down somewhere in the building—is necessary, it cannot, and should not ever, replace having a weekly sit down. (para. 1)

Moncho's advice is valuable for genetic counseling supervision, regardless of the site's volume or intensity.

Attend genetic counseling program supervisor meetings. Genetic counseling programs conduct periodic sessions with supervisors to review program expectations, provide updates about program changes, and discuss anonymized feedback from former students' evaluations of their experiences at the site (Hendrickson et al., 2002).

Conduct student orientations. Both genetic counseling programs and rotation sites can hold orientation sessions for students to learn what the rotations and supervision entail (Hendrickson et al., 2002).

Closing Thoughts

Anticipating and addressing critical elements of the supervision experience contribute to developing a strong working relationship that promotes positive supervision processes and outcomes. The strategies described in this chapter may help you develop and maintain a "bifocal" lens, viewing supervision through both supervisors' and students' eyes. Given the time-limited nature of most genetic counseling student supervision, the more things you can do to "hit the ground running," the further students may be able to advance in their professional development.

Learning Activities

Most learning activities can be adapted for dyad or small group discussions or for written exercises. Time estimates are provided for discussions, but additional time should be allotted for large group processing.

Activity 3.1 Working Alliance Factors

With a partner, create a list of supervisor personal qualities and traits you believe contribute to an optimal supervisory working alliance.

Then, using this list, identify three to five supervisor qualities that each of you regards as particularly important in the supervisory relationship.

Are there qualities you find/would find challenging in your own provision of supervision?

Estimated time: 15 minutes

Note: This activity can be expanded by asking participants to also identify student qualities and traits that contribute to an optimal supervisory working alliance.

Activity 3.2 Prepping for Supervision—Getting Started

List three things you typically do (or would do if you have not been a supervisor) to prepare for starting a supervision relationship with a student:

1.

2.

3.

Share your list with a partner or in small groups.

Estimated time: 20 minutes

Note: This activity can be modified and then completed by students to help prepare them to start a supervision relationship.

Activity 3.3 Prepping for Supervision— Anticipating Student Questions

List the top five questions you would want to ask a student before beginning supervision with them:

1.

2.

3.

4.

5.

Share your list with a partner or in small groups.

Estimated time: 15 minutes

Activity 3.4 Challenging Student Questions

Using Appendix 3A, identify three or four student questions you find/would find challenging to answer. What makes each question challenging for you?

Share your responses with a partner or in small groups.

Estimated time: 20 minutes

Activity 3.5 Supervision Information Statement/ Agreement

Prepare a two-page, single-spaced statement you could give to a student at the beginning of your supervisory relationship. Refer to Table 3.1 for elements to consider including in your statement. If you are a student, pretend you are a certified genetic counselor and "make up" information about where you work/specialty area.

Hints: The statement should be *user-friendly* (e.g., descriptions should be stated simply, with clear terminology and definitions). There should be good transitions between topics; side headings can help with transitions. Be sure to give your statement a title. You may wish to review the examples in Appendixes 3C and 3D. McCarthy and LeRoy (2009) also provide an example. The questions listed in Appendix 3A may stimulate your thinking about content you would like to include.

Note: This activity can be expanded by asking participants to identify questions from Appendix 3A they believe they have addressed in their information statement. The activity can also be expanded by having participants role play presenting and discussing their statement with a partner who plays the role of a student.

Appendix 3A
Genetic Counseling Student Questions About Supervision

These questions include both those that students may ask directly and those that may remain unspoken. They represent questions and concerns of novice and more advanced students.

Supervisor–Student Relationship

- Am I going to get along with you?
- Are you a tough supervisor?
- Will you like me?
- Are you going to be nice? Are you going to be mean to me?
- Will we have similar styles?
- How can we co-counsel as a team? How can I pass it back to you? How would you like to format sessions where we take a team approach?
- How can I make sure you know that I'm invested?

Supervisor Prior Knowledge of Student

- What have you heard about me?
- What did other supervisors tell you about me?

Student Prior Knowledge of Supervisor

- What is your reputation as a supervisor?
- What were other students' experiences with you?
- Have you had conflicts with other students in the past?

Supervisor Characteristics and Styles

- What are your credentials?
- What is your background?
- Are you qualified?
- How much experience do you have as a supervisor?
- How do you feel about supervising?
- Are you a flexible supervisor, or do you like things done a certain way?
- What is your personality type or style (calm/chill vs. formal/strict)?
- What is your supervisor style?
- Are you able to appreciate counseling styles that differ from yours?
- Would you modify your style?
- Do you remember what it was like to be a student?

Supervision Structure and Processes

- Will our supervision focus on case prep? Clients? My professional development?
- What are your typical supervision techniques during a session?

- What can and can't I talk about in supervision?
- How often will we meet?
- How long will our meetings be?

Genetic Counseling Service Provision—Structure and Processes

- What are your expectations of roles in sessions—what will I need to do?
- How much of the session will I be asked to do?
- What will happen in the room in general (or in the session if the appointment is telehealth)?
- How do you behave during the session—do you sit behind me and take notes or sit beside me?
- What is going to happen in the session with the client if correction is needed?
- What is going to happen in the session with the client if an issue/challenge arises?
- Will there be time before the session to discuss approach?
- How should I approach a case that I haven't encountered before?
- Is it possible to have an extended time frame if I need to go over the scheduled time?
- Is it ok if I observe? Are there opportunities for observation throughout the rotation?
- Do you expect me to go in by myself at some point in the rotation? Will there be an opportunity to counsel alone? Option for independent session? Can I do full sessions?
- Will I be pushed to do things I'm not comfortable with?
- If there is an unexpected add-on client I didn't prepare for, will I be expected to see them?

The "Step-In"

- How "hands on" are you going to be in sessions? Do you jump in/hang back?

- How do I get help from you when needed in session?
- How will you stop me if I'm wrong?
- What signs will you give me to let me know how it's going/how I'm doing?
- How do I interrupt you/take back a session?
- How should I interpret a jump-in by you?

Case Preparation/Follow-Up

- What expectations and/or preferences do you have for case prep?
- How much prep do I need to do for cases?
- How much time would I have to prep for cases?
- Are there any special things specific to this clinic that I should be paying close attention to in the chart?
- What can I expect from you in terms of willingness to look at my prep for a case?
- Do you write client letters or clinic notes to document your cases? Which would you like me to do?
- How soon should I submit letters?
- How many hours do you anticipate me spending on clinical pre- and post-prep work? How long do you think I should typically spend on a case prep?

Flexibility

- Will there be flexibility with my counseling style and involvement?
- How much freedom will I have to explore my own counseling style?
- Will there be flexibility in the rotation regarding progress, learning, and managing roles?
- How much latitude do I have to deviate from the plan for a client?

Supervisor Expectations

- What are the site-specific expectations for students?
- What and how much do you specifically expect of me by the end of the rotation?
- What expectations do you have for my involvement in sessions?
- Are your expectations reasonable?
- Do you have specific goals for me? What are they?
- What do you expect of me regarding deadlines?
- What do you expect regarding case follow-up?
- What are the expectations for a typical day?

Feedback and Evaluation

- How do I receive feedback?
- When do I receive feedback?
- What's the turnaround time for feedback on letters?
- Where do I receive feedback?
- What are your feedback and debriefing methods?
- How critical are you going to be?
- Will I be quizzed? Will you try to "catch me/call me out" for not knowing things?
- How will I find out if I'm doing something wrong?
- When can I speak up in response to feedback?
- What is your impression of my skill set?
- What will you think I need to work on? Be allowed to do?
- How will I be evaluated?
- Is there a formal midterm evaluation for the rotation?
- What information will you use to evaluate me?
- What are you going to write in my evaluation that you won't tell me?
- Who do you talk with about my performance?

Client Population

- What is the socioeconomic status of clients at this site?
- What are the clients' backgrounds?
- What type of client encounters will we have?
- What types of cases should I expect?

Logistics

- Will we meet to discuss goals before the first day of clinic?
- How do I get there? Will there be parking?
- What technology will we use for telehealth visits and how will I access it?
- Where should I meet you?
- How many days per week do you expect me in clinic? Which days?
- How long each day? What hours do I need to be here?
- Is there a scheduled time for lunch?
- What should I do in the event I am sick, running late, etc.? Who do I contact and how?
- What is the best way to contact you?
- What is your availability during the week?
- What is the clinic structure?
- Are there any extra projects associated with this rotation?
- What would you like me to be doing in my downtime?
- What is the rotation schedule?
- What is the pace? Will I be rushed? Is time a big concern?
- How many clients are there per day?
- How long are sessions?
- What practices, protocols should I follow?
- How do we document clinic notes? Templates? Created ourselves?
- What are we doing on the first day?

- Will you assign me clients, will I choose clients, or will I see every client with you?
- How do changes in client/schedule get communicated to students?

Interacting with Other Staff

- Who are the staff, and what are their roles?
- Who will I be interacting/working with?
- How do interactions with the rest of the medical staff occur?
- How can and should I communicate with staff?
- When can I/should I communicate with staff?
- How should I present information to the physician?
- Will other health care providers be giving feedback on my skills?
- When and how should I (as a student) communicate changes in the schedule?

Resources

- Are there any important resources you use that I should get for this rotation?
- What materials do you recommend I read and understand before starting?
- How do you feel about the importance of visual aids/flipbook? Do you have any specific visual aid recommendations?
- What sources do you use for risk numbers? Where would you prefer I get my numbers from?

Appendix 3B
Genetic Counselor Supervisor Questions
About Students

The following questions include both those supervisors may ask directly and those that may remain unspoken. Some questions are particularly relevant for students who have had prior supervised training experiences.

Student–Supervisor Relationship

- What is your image of an ideal supervision relationship?
- How can I be most helpful to you as a supervisor?
- How will you feel eliciting help/advice from me?
- How would you approach and address any conflict that arises between us?
- What is something you would like me to know about *you*?
- What is something you would like to know about *me*?
- What is something you do for fun?

Student Characteristics and Styles

- Here are descriptions of four supervisory styles. . . .Which one(s) do you prefer?
- What has worked well for you in prior supervision relationships?
- What has been challenging for you in prior supervision relationships?
- How would you describe your cultural background? Are there aspects of your identity that you would like me to know more about? (See also Chapter 4.)
- What skills from a prior rotation(s) will be translatable?

- What prior experiences, if any, have you had with the types of clients seen at this clinic?
- How will you communicate in a session that you need me to jump in?
- How much co-counseling do you expect from me?
- For emotional genetic counseling sessions, what kind of support do you want from me?
- What type of debrief is helpful to you?

Student Expectations

- What are two goals you have for this rotation?
- What do you think will be most rewarding about this rotation?
- What do you think will be most challenging about this rotation?
- What do you think will be the most prominent skill you will learn?
- How does this rotation fit into your career goals?

Feedback and Evaluation

- What was the most important positive feedback you received at your last rotation?
- What was the most important corrective feedback you received at your last rotation?
- How do you want to obtain feedback?
- What fears do you have regarding feedback?
- How do you usually respond to positive feedback? To corrective feedback?
- How will you handle feedback that is confusing to you?

Appendix 3C
Sample Information Sheet

Template

Name
Office Location
Desk Phone
Mobile
Fax
Email
Work Hours/Days of Supervisor
Preferred Method(s) of Contact
Supervisor's Clinics (with times and locations)
Overall Description of Rotation
Rotation-Specific Learning Objectives
Rotation-Specific Expectations:

- Communication
- Time Commitment/Caseload
- Other Requirements

Other Learning Opportunities Available on This Rotation

Example

Name
Office Location
Desk Phone
Mobile
Email

Work Hours/Days of Supervisor
  Monday through Friday, 8 a.m.–5 p.m.
Preferred Method(s) of Contact
  Email

Supervisor's Clinics (with Times and Locations)
- General Genetics Clinic
  - Monday afternoons, Outpatient Genetics Clinic (Building A, Level 2)
- Hereditary Cancer Clinic
  - Tuesday and Thursday mornings, Oncology Outpatient clinic (Building B, Level 4)
- Genetic Counseling Only Clinic
  - 1st and 3rd Wednesday afternoons, Telehealth Center (Building A, Level 4)
  - 2nd and 4th Friday mornings, Outpatient Genetics Clinic (Building A, Level 2)

Overall Description of Rotation

During this rotation, you will have the opportunity to see clients for general genetics (both kids and adults) as well as for hereditary cancer (mostly adults). For General Genetics clinic, we will be working collaboratively with a clinical geneticist. Depending on the point in your training, you will have the opportunity to take on all General Genetics roles including case management and follow-up.

Rotation-Specific Learning Objectives
- Incorporate electronic medical records into case preparation and participation in the case
- Demonstrate knowledge of etiology, testing options, outcomes, and cancer risks
- Develop a differential diagnosis for a patient referred to General Genetics clinic
- Obtain a targeted family and medical history
- Become familiar with risk factors that are indicative of a hereditary cancer syndrome
- Provide psychosocial counseling to families and provide resources for ongoing support as needed
- Become familiar with testing options and be able to describe testing options to patients and families

- Complete follow-up with families as indicated
- Coordinate genetic testing and communicate results to families

Rotation-Specific Expectations
- Communication
  - **Before the rotation**: Contact me the week before the rotation to set up an initial meeting. Bring to this meeting your goals for the rotation. We will discuss supervision as well as logistics of the rotation at this initial meeting.
  - **During the Rotation**: At our initial meeting, we will set up a weekly meeting where we will discuss your progress, cases you have seen for that week, and which cases you would like to participate in the following week. In addition to these regular meetings, we will meet just after clinic whenever possible to reflect and provide feedback on the cases you have seen that day. The day before a client you will be seeing is scheduled, you will need to email any case preparation materials or questions you have related to the client. If I do not receive this email, you will not be able to see the client. If you have a lot of questions or concerns before a case, we can schedule a time to meet before seeing the client.
  - **End of the Rotation**: We will meet the week after the end of the rotation to go over your final evaluation.
- Time Commitment/Caseload
  - Minimum of 2 clients per week, but more are encouraged if possible.
- Documentation
  - I will complete all case evaluations electronically and review them with you after each case or at the end of a clinic.
  - Case logs/summaries must be completed within a week of seeing the case. Email me when a case is ready for my review in the online documentation system.
- Other Requirements
  - We will be using the electronic medical record system for case prep and documentation. If you have not used it before, let me know so we can review at our first meeting.

Other Learning Opportunities Available on This Rotation
- Case Conference—Mondays at 8 a.m.
  - Genetic counselors and geneticists meet to review cases. You are welcome to attend this meeting each week.
  - If there is a case you see that is being presented, you can take the lead on this presentation.

Appendix 3D
Sample Information Agreement

Welcome to Supervision

Purpose

The purpose of this document is to align our expectations for what supervision will include and how it will be carried out, and address questions you may have about our supervision experience. After reading this document, questions may arise, which I encourage you to address with me.

My Background

I am an American Board of Genetic Counseling certified genetic counselor, licensed in this state. I completed my master's degree in the XXX genetic program at XXX. I have XXX years of post-degree experience, primarily providing prenatal genetic counseling. I have worked at this clinic for XX years. Regarding my supervision experience, I have supervised XXX genetic counseling students and XXX medical residents. I attend supervision trainings annually.

Practical Issues

We will meet weekly in my office for 30-minute, mandatory individual supervision sessions (to be scheduled prior to your first week in clinic). If you anticipate being unable to attend a supervision meeting and/or clinic, you are responsible for making alternative arrangements in advance. In an emergency, please notify me as soon as possible. I will give you my contact information at our first meeting.

Supervision Process

Supervision is an interactive process intended to improve your genetic counseling skills, increase your professional self-identity, monitor your provision of services, assist you to make independent professional decisions, and enhance your ability to critically examine your own practice, thus encouraging self-supervision skills.

We will discuss cases prior to each clinic, together determine appropriate interventions, and decide which interventions you will be responsible for conducting. During our supervision interactions, you will have the opportunity to ask questions, explore alternative interventions, address ethical concerns, and engage in a feedback process related to your rotation activities.

My typical approach to supervision conversations involves a mix of evocative and directive teaching. I also use consultant, counselor, and evaluator approaches as appropriate. I will explain these approaches to you during our first meeting.

I am ultimately responsible for the services you provide, as well as for assisting you in your professional development through activities that include goal setting, feedback, and evaluations. You can expect to receive timely verbal and written feedback on your clinical performance and progress. You are responsible for adhering to agency policies (see attachment), being on time for rotation and supervision activities, being prepared for cases, documenting service provision, preparing follow-up letters, and following through on all assignments and recommendations. You are also responsible for coming prepared to actively participate in supervision, remaining open and responsive to feedback, self-evaluating, disclosing important information, asking for assistance as needed, and being willing to take learning risks.

Issues of cultural identity, as they affect our work and your work with clients, are an integral part of supervision. My policy on discrimination based on race, ethnicity, gender, sexual orientation, or disability complies with genetic counseling profession standards, and that is zero tolerance. If you have concerns or difficulty related to any of these types of discrimination, I intend to foster a supportive environment for you to safely discuss your thoughts with me directly, or with an alternative person, should the need arise.

Supervision Benefits and Risks

Possible beneficial outcomes of your supervision experience include meeting rotation objectives (see attachment) and increased confidence about your genetic counseling knowledge and skills.

Supervision can become emotionally intense at times, and you may feel some level of discomfort in being challenged to think and feel more deeply about your counseling knowledge and skills. Remember, the ultimate goal is to grow as a professional and responsible genetic counselor.

Evaluation/Due Process

I will provide you with ongoing oral and written feedback throughout this rotation. A formal written evaluation will be conducted upon completion. Evaluation criteria include your performance in the setting, meeting the set of objectives for this rotation, and an assessment of your progress attaining skills necessary to practice as a genetic counselor. A formal written evaluation of my supervision will be solicited from you at the end of the rotation. If at any time you are concerned about your supervision or the evaluation process, please discuss this with me. If we are unable to resolve your concerns, or you find it difficult to speak with me directly, you are urged to discuss them with the director of your genetic counseling graduate program.

Legal/Ethical Issues

Supervision is not intended to provide personal counseling for you. I strongly encourage you to seek counseling if personal concerns arise. In general, the content of our supervision sessions is confidential. I will share my evaluations of your development with your program director. Formal written evaluations are retained by your program director. You can expect that I will not discuss your progress with your fellow students. Limits to confidentiality include, but are not limited to, treatment of a client that violates legal or ethical standards established by this clinic, your program/institution, and/or the genetic counseling profession.

Addendum
After we discuss this document at our first supervision meeting, please write any statements you would like to add (You may attach additional pages if necessary):

Statement of Agreement
I read and had the opportunity to ask questions about the information contained in this document.

_____   _____

(Supervisor's Signature)   Date

_____   _____

(Student's Signature)   Date

4

Culturally Engaged Supervision

IAN M. MACFARLANE AND

KRISTA REDLINGER-GROSSE

Objectives

- Describe cultural engagement in supervision.
- Articulate theory regarding cultural engagement in supervision.
- Identify ways culture can create opportunities and barriers in supervision.
- Provide strategies for incorporating identity discussions in genetic counseling supervision and for managing client biases when students are involved.

Introduction

The field of genetic counseling is ever changing, not only in scientific and technological advances but also in the diversity of the profession. The principles of justice, equity, diversity, and inclusion (JEDI) have become a professional priority (National Society of Genetic Counselors [NSGC], 2021); with this comes the need

Both authors contributed equally to the development of this chapter and consider themselves co-first authors.

to focus on JEDI efforts in training, specifically in supervision practices to support culturally diverse genetic counseling students (Carmichael et al., 2021). Given the lifelong nature of the work, cultural engagement is a goal in the Reciprocal-Engagement Model of Supervision (REM-S; Wherley et al. 2015; see Chapter 1, this volume) and a defined competency in genetic counseling supervision (Eubanks Higgins et al., 2013). One of the REM-S goals states that supervisors "integrate personal and professional, and cultural context into the supervision relationship and decisions" (Wherley et al., 2015, p. 710); and Eubanks Higgins et al. (2013) describe competent supervisors as those who "explore their own cultural identity and how this identity affects their values and beliefs about counseling and supervision" (p. 53). As JEDI efforts increase in the genetic counseling field (NSGC, 2021), culturally engaged supervision becomes a more relevant and important focus of supervision training.

It can be challenging to broach the topics of culture and identity with students. These are sensitive topics central to who we and our supervisees are. Thus, there can be a temptation to shy away from discussing them openly because of the potential to say or do the wrong thing or the sense that they are "beyond the scope" of the supervisory role. What we sometimes fail to remember, however, are the opportunities an open dialogue about cultural differences (and similarities!) can bring to the relationship. These opportunities include

- modeling how to address culture and identity with clients through parallel processes;
- demonstrating to students that we recognize the importance of these issues and are willing to engage despite the possibility of missteps;
- opening ourselves to learning about inclusive ways to approach our work as genetic counselors that might improve our practice;

- supporting students, especially those from underrepresented backgrounds who may not offer up their culture and identity without invitation; and
- creating the potential for a deeper and more meaningful interpersonal connection with students (and future colleagues).

Important Terminology

The discussion of culturally engaged supervision must begin with a careful definition of terms we use in this chapter. The language around culture, identity, power, and privilege is continually evolving, and we recognize these words may be supplanted by terms that are more popular, more inclusive, or more nuanced. We celebrate the evolution of this language. We hope the terms we use continue to convey respect and careful thought, but the odds are that at least some of the language in this chapter will age poorly. We strongly encourage you to stay up to date with shifting terminology and carefully consider the impact of words as you engage with students, colleagues, clients, and the public. All that said, what follows is a brief summary of a rich literature on a sprawling, multifaceted construct.

Culture

Culture must be considered broadly in order to appreciate the multiple interweaving "complex cultural influences" that contribute to an individual's identity (P. Hays, 1996, p. 332). Hays (1996) proposed the ADDRESSING model as a "transcultural-specific perspective" that draws attention to nine cultural factors warranting consideration and appreciation in understanding supervisors'/supervisees' intersecting cultural identities and backgrounds (P. Hays, 1996, p. 334). Box 4.1 contains an explanation of this acronym.

BOX 4.1 The ADDRESSING Model

Age and generational influences
Developmental disabilities
Disabilities acquired later in life
Religion and spiritual orientation
Ethnic and racial identity
Socioeconomic status
Sexual orientation
Indigenous heritage
National origin
Gender

Source: Hays, P. (1996). Addressing the complexities of counseling and gender in counseling. *Journal of Counseling and Development, 74*, 332–338.

The ADDRESSING model is not intended to be exhaustive but, rather, to provide a starting point to consider cultural influences in a more integrated way and begin self-reflection on important contextual influences and potential areas of bias and assumptions for the student and supervisor, and also to work toward a more identity-conscious supervisory relationship (Talusan, 2021).

Cultural Competence

Cultural competence is the most prominent and commonly used term to describe the ability to work productively across cultural differences. There are various claims as to who coined the term, but it appeared in nursing, social work, and counseling psychology in the late 1970s and early 1980s (e.g., Gallegos, 1982; Leininger, 1978; Sue et al., 1982), moved into other aspects of health care in the 1990s (e.g., Campinha-Bacote, 1994; Purnell & Paulanka, 1998), and was incorporated into professional codes of conduct and educational requirements for training programs across health care around 2000 (Fisher-Borne et al., 2015). Early models of cultural competence outlined stages of development. For example, Cross (1988) describes six stages: cultural destructiveness, covert discrimination, cultural blindness, cultural precompetency, cultural competence, and cultural proficiency. Later models emphasize domains rather than stages. For example, Sue's (2001) multidimensional model of cultural competence has three dimensions: components (knowledge, skills, and attitudes), foci (individual, professional, organizational, and societal), and cultural-specific attributes (African American, Asian American, Latino American, Native American, and European American). Purnell's (2002) model has 12 domains (e.g., family roles, communication, and spirituality) in which practitioners can be unconsciously incompetent, consciously incompetent, consciously competent, or unconsciously competent.

Definitions of cultural competence vary, but they typically center on the ability to accurately assess cultural issues relevant to practice and adapt interventions accordingly. Although typically applied to individuals, the concept has been adapted to organizations and systems (for a systematic review, see L. Anderson et al., 2003). Criticisms of this term largely center around the idea of competence being an endpoint and that if a specified amount of information can be learned, competence is ensured (e.g., Camphina-Bacote, 2018). Additional criticisms include lack of attention to systemic issues, emphasis on knowledge rather than process, potential to stereotype people based on their identities, and focus on practitioner comfort (e.g., Beagen, 2018; Camphina-Bacote, 2018; Fisher-Borne et al., 2015). Although many models of cultural competence explicitly include ongoing development and a sense that competence is never truly achieved, this term is losing favor because of the implied stagnation.

Cultural Humility

Tervalon and Murray-Garcia (1998) proposed *cultural humility* as an alternative to cultural competence. Cultural humility emphasizes the continuous, dynamic, and introspective nature of incorporating cultural understanding into health care practices. Humility is meant to underscore the need for practitioners to foreground client needs, protect against the tendency to apply stereotypes, and view cultural understanding as a process rather than an achievement. A cultural humility approach emphasizes ongoing self-reflection to identify practitioners' own dynamic and evolving biases, assumptions, and worldviews. Some scholars (e.g., Danso, 2016) have argued that the tenets of cultural humility are not particularly distinct from cultural competence and the term is gaining traction largely due to "semantic appeal" rather than innovation. Others have argued that instead of replacing competence, cultural humility is best situated as complementary to competence (e.g., Yancu & Farmer, 2017).

Cultural Engagement

Our preferred term, and one we use throughout this chapter, is *cultural engagement*. We were introduced to this term by Dr. Maria Morales as we prepared to co-lead a supervisor workshop on diversity, equity, and inclusion (DEI) issues in genetic counseling supervision, and we have championed it since. To us, this more active term places the onus on practitioners to put energy into this process. If cultural competence emphasizes the "what" and humility emphasizes the "how," engagement can be the overarching drive to push forward on JEDI efforts. Engagement also carries the implied question of "With whom?" It is critical to engage with our students, our clients, our colleagues, and ourselves as we do this work; in doing so, cultural engagement bridges competence's emphasis on the "other" and humility's emphasis on the self. Although Danso's (2016) critique of making decisions based on semantic appeal applies to us as well, our stance is that words used to convey ideas matter more than just a shorthand for the underlying theory.

Additional Terms

Other alternatives for this process of exploring culture include cultural responsiveness (Sue et al., 1991), cultural safety (Papps &

Ramsden, 1996), cultural compatibility (Camphina-Bacote, 2018), transnational competence (Koehn & Swick, 2006), and identity-conscious (Talusan, 2021), all which have strengths and limitations.

Foundations in Theory and Research

Limited research concerns the role of culture and identity in genetic counseling supervision. In one study, supervisors' multicultural awareness and knowledge predicted their ability to discern culturally appropriate versus inappropriate responses to a hypothetical scenario (Lee et al., 2009). Although no other studies link JEDI skills or awareness to supervision outcomes, several point to the need for increased training on these topics. In one study, supervisors had difficulty identifying strategies specific to culturally engaged (competent) supervision (Suguitan et al., 2019). Genetic counseling students who identify as racial or ethnic minorities have reported feeling isolated in their programs due to their identity (Carmichael et al., 2020; Schoonveld et al., 2007). They have also reported experiencing discomfort in their clinical rotations due to racism and microaggressions from patients, health team members, and their supervisors (Carmichael et al., 2021). Students report race and ethnicity may be addressed in supervision when the focus is on student–patient dynamics, but generally not in student–supervisor dynamics (Dewey et al., 2021). Carmichael and colleagues (2021) also highlighted how incorporating conversations about cultural identity into the supervisory relationship has the potential to help students see their identities as positive resources at their disposal, such as their ability to switch cultural frames when interacting with clients.

The counseling and psychotherapy supervision literatures are more extensive in terms of JEDI issues, including specific calls for supervisors to address areas of diversity between themselves and their supervisees (e.g., Barnett & Molzon, 2014; D. Hays & Chang, 2003). Numerous models recommend supervisors assess their own and their supervisees' stages of identity development (e.g., Cook, 1994). These models often focus on a single element of identity (predominantly race/ethnicity), although there are more recent movements toward more multifaceted and intersectional frameworks (e.g., Ancis & Ladany, 2010; Peters, 2017). From the many summaries of best practices and recommendations for supervisors (e.g., Estrada et al., 2004; Norman, 2015; Wong et al., 2013), we extracted the following consistent guidelines:

- Establish trust and safety through a strong supervisory working alliance.
- Initiate open conversations about culture and diversity early in the relationship.
- Engage in ongoing self-assessment to explore your strengths, growth areas, blind spots, and countertransference related to aspects of JEDI.
- Revisit conversations about culture throughout the supervisory relationship.
- Expect missteps and misunderstandings to occur, and be ready to repair relationships when they do.

Elements of these guidelines are evident in genetic counseling supervision literature (e.g., Carmichael et al., 2021; Dewey et al., 2021; Suguitan et al., 2019; Wherley et al., 2015).

Culturally Engaged Supervision: Applications and Strategies

Culturally engaged supervision is an ongoing process built on intentional practice. As we discuss strategies and applications, we include a scenario to go along with each. These scenarios are based on examples taken from workshops we have conducted, stories shared by supervisors and students, and genetic counseling literature. Although grounded in real experiences, the scenarios are fictional. Some may be challenging to read, especially if you have similarly experienced or witnessed microaggressions, racism, and/or cultural insensitivity in your training, supervision, or practice. The following strategies may help you pace yourself through this material:

> *Engage with cultural humility.* Cultural self-awareness and appreciation are critical elements in building supervisory relationships.
>
> *Be open and nonjudgmental.* Because cultural engagement is challenging, this work comes with fears and expectations that we will make mistakes along the way. It is important to remember that mistakes are normative in the growth process. As Skyler Stef Jarvi (Former Director of Education for the University of Minnesota's Office of Equity and Diversity) would often say in trainings, "If you're not messing up, you're not showing up" (S. Stef Jarvi, personal communication, June 17, 2020). We encourage our students to take chances in sessions and trust themselves to grow from mistakes. So, let's model this process by being open to the process and nonjudgmental with ourselves and others.
>
> *Self-assess.* Self-reflective practice is necessary for culturally engaged supervision. Take time along the way to self-assess and engage in consultation and supervision about this process for support.
>
> *Come back to this chapter.* Cultural engagement is a lifelong practice, and we discover new things each time we recommit to our development in this area. You will continue to have experiences that may unlock new insights or questions about engaging with others, so make time to regularly revisit your perspectives.

To facilitate your engagement and learning with each of these scenarios, we offer questions to guide your reflections and to assist you in focusing on one issue rather than getting lost or overwhelmed by potential supervision concerns. We recognize, however, that with each scenario there may be many opportunities for cultural engagement. We also acknowledge from the outset that the scenarios largely revolve around race and ethnicity. This was a conscious decision to provide some continuity across scenarios and reduce the number of variables to consider when building a repertoire of strategies. We do not mean to suggest race/ethnicity is the only area of identity in which culturally engaged supervision is applicable or needed. The strategies herein are broad enough to work with many forms of diversity, and we provide several additional scenarios at the end of the chapter that highlight other marginalized identities to provide space to start applying the lessons of the chapter in other contexts.

Starting Point: Cultural Self-Awareness

Culturally engaged supervision starts from within. Internal self-awareness "represents how clearly we see our own values, passions, aspirations, fit with our environment, reactions (including thoughts, feelings, behaviors, strengths, and weakness), and impact on others" (Eurich, 2018, para 5). A greater sense of internal self-awareness around culture can increase your cultural perspective taking or cultural empathy.

Cultural self-awareness can be understood as "an individual's metacognitive understanding of culture's influence on the self. It encompasses an understanding of the link between oneself and cultural experience" (Lu & Wan, 2018, p. 823). Developing your cultural self-awareness will provide a clearer sense of how your own cultural experiences have shaped you, specifically your values and behaviors that can inform biases and assumptions you bring to the supervisory relationship. When left unchecked, implicit biases can lead to blind spots and, in the worst cases, unacknowledged disparaging comments in supervision. The following scenario illustrates unexamined culture:

Scenario 1

Jon has been a supervisor for more than 10 years and has thoroughly enjoyed his work with genetic counseling students. He recently participated in a DEI workshop through his department and heard from other science, technology, engineering, and mathematics (STEM) graduate students about their challenging experiences of working with White, male faculty. He left the workshop feeling unsettled and wondering how many times he had "stuck his foot in his mouth" with his supervisees, specifically those who came from different backgrounds than his own. Jon grew up in a small, rural town where "these things" were just not talked about, let alone supported. He questioned, "Where do I even begin?"

In this scenario, Jon is beginning to be aware of an opportunity (and need) to grow in his cultural self-awareness.

Reflection Questions for Readers: What similarities and differences do you see between yourself and Jon as a supervisor? What do you see as next steps for Jon in growing his cultural self-awareness? How do you anticipate growth in cultural self-awareness may assist Jon in working toward more culturally engaged supervision?

Jon's participation in department DEI work suggests he has some interest in the topic and some awareness of its importance. He has even started to reflect on past experiences and had moments of feeling "unsettled" when he wonders how he may have unintentionally said or done something that negatively impacted students. Thus, Jon is beginning to gain some insight into his need to do his own work in the DEI or JEDI space. At this starting point, Jon's next step may be to begin doing some internal work and name his identities and how they place him in positions of privilege (e.g., White, male working in the STEM field, and educated). With this increased awareness, Jon may be able to further explore and uncover ways these identities present growth opportunities in working with students who are similar to and different from him.

As mentioned previously, the ADDRESSING framework is a place to start examining our many cultural aspects and how they intersect. To facilitate this self-exploration, Appendix 4A contains a worksheet we developed to walk you through the ADDRESSING framework. We recommend that you revisit this worksheet periodically. Just as the work of culturally engaged supervision is ongoing, so is the work of understanding our own identities and the impact of our work. For example, the biases and assumptions we hold based on our identities, as well as our willingness to disclose (or not) our identities, influence how we manage potential supervision dynamics such as countertransference (see Chapter 14).

Entry Points: Communication

Because starting the conversation about culture and identity is often the most difficult part, we typically ease into it by building off another topic. This strategy allows for building trust and safety in the supervisory relationship without jumping quickly into vulnerable and potentially activating topics. There is no single way to safely bring culture and identity into discussions with your students. The following are just a few possible methods for foregrounding culture and identity. We encourage you to bring these issues up regularly and in multiple ways to enrich the supervisory relationship.

Communication of Expectations

Embed the conversation of culture and identity into a broader discussion about communication processes and styles. Rotations often start with communication of expectations, so including how you and your student are going to communicate is a natural offshoot (see Chapter 3). Communication styles and patterns are highly influenced by culture, but we often assume everyone communicates the same way we do. This assumption can lead to misinterpretations by supervisors and/or students. Consider, for example, a supervisor who communicates directly while their student communicates indirectly. The student may experience the supervisor as hostile or aggressive, whereas the supervisor may experience the student as disinterested or passive. If you can identify how you typically communicate and share this information with students, you can start conversations about how they prefer to communicate and how the two of you can best communicate with each other. We believe developing a shared understanding of how each of you approaches the work and making modifications to your usual patterns of behavior to facilitate a working alliance are the heart of a culturally engaged approach to supervision. Demonstrating thoughtfulness about how you and your student communicate signals to the student that you recognize differences between the two of you that will impact the work. Moreover, if you show willingness to be flexible, this will likely increase the student's trust in you (provided you follow through on what you agree to). The process of exploring communication styles and co-creating communication norms can serve as a model for negotiating numerous aspects of your work together.

To facilitate this conversation, Appendix 4B contains a brief worksheet we developed to help you identify where you fall on several domains of communication. It also serves as a useful way to start conversations with your student about communication. We recommend you fill this out and reflect on how your communication style affects how you supervise students. We also recommend you discuss communication styles explicitly with your students, perhaps by sending your completed worksheet to them during your initial email interactions along with a blank copy for them to complete. You could even ask graduate program(s) leadership you work with to have their students collectively complete the worksheet as part of a class activity. Discussing similarities and differences on the sheet with your student can be an excellent early conversation that naturally leads into talking about other dynamics that might affect your work together (e.g., identity statuses).

Think about communication dynamics as you read the following scenario:

Scenario 2

Andrea is a first-generation college graduate who moved to the United States with her parents when she was 10 years old. Andrea eagerly began her rotation with Jessica, the lead supervisor. Jessica had instructed Andrea to come to the first day of clinic prepared to share her past clinical experiences, rotation-specific goals, and expectations for Jessica and supervision. After orienting Andrea to the clinic and staff, Jessica and Andrea sat down to get to know one another and discuss Andrea's responses to Jessica's questions. To Jessica's surprise (and disappointment), Andrea fumbled through responses with short and quick answers. When Jessica asked if she had any questions for her, Andrea answered, "No" and looked at her with a neutral expression. Jessica concluded that Andrea clearly was uninterested in being in clinic and worried about how to keep her engaged for the remainder of the rotation.

In this situation, expectations around communication appear to differ between Jessica and Andrea.

Reflection Questions for Readers: What can you infer about the communication expectations that Jessica holds for Andrea? What are some potential cultural explanations/hypotheses for Andrea's brief answers and communication style? How would you broach a conversation about communication expectations with Andrea?

You may have noticed Jessica seemed to expect a prepared response to her questions. She also seemed to equate having questions (and the sharing of them) as a measure of interest in the rotation. Andrea may come from a culture with more hierarchical communication, where offering expectations about how supervision would unfold could be considered rude, aggressive, or dismissive of her supervisor's role. Andrea may also have a more relational communication style and find it jarring to jump into tasks immediately before rapport has been established. Andrea may view asking questions as a marker of being unprepared, and she does not want to give a poor impression on the first day. There are myriad potential explanations for why this exchange happened the way it did, and the conclusions Jessica draws quickly move to a poor reflection on Andrea. First impressions are difficult to shift, so this conversation may set the tone for the rest of the rotation. This is why conversations about communication styles and expectations at the outset can be so valuable.

Take the initiative to model vulnerability in these conversations and invite feedback on how things are going throughout the rotation. Given the power we hold as supervisors, the onus is on us to demonstrate we can be trusted in these challenging conversations by listening carefully, owning our mistakes as we make them, and working collaboratively with students to shape the supervisory relationship.

Communication of Feedback

Communication is especially important in the delivery of feedback to your student. Students often find feedback both the most rewarding and the most challenging aspect of supervision (MacFarlane et al., 2016; see Chapter 7, this volume), and stress around feedback tends to be higher for early rotation students. Being in the position of power in the relationship due to the evaluation inherent in supervision, we need to pay particular attention to how we communicate feedback. Feedback should come from a place of helping students reach competence and become independent practitioners. Despite this noble intention, we must own the impact of our feedback and acknowledge that sometimes it will not live up to these goals. When done appropriately, feedback can be an entry point to deepening cultural understanding, but it can also erect barriers if not handled well.

Consider the following scenario in which a supervisor's attempts at feedback seem to have caused a rupture in the relationship:

Scenario 3

Kyla is just over halfway through her rotation with her supervisor Taylor. Thus far, Kyla is doing an adequate job. Her skills are about what one would expect for a student at her level of experience, and Taylor gave her a fairly positive mid-rotation evaluation. During the past week, however, Taylor noticed Kyla is communicating less and keeps her answers short when directly addressed. This is particularly surprising to Taylor, as she listed professionalism on her evaluation as the primary area Kyla needed to improve. Specifically, Taylor asked her to show more enthusiasm for the work, ask more questions, share more about what she's thinking when she makes mistakes, and show more appreciation for the detailed feedback Taylor provides. Kyla identifies as a different race and religion than Taylor, and although there was a brief discussion of these differences at the beginning of the rotation, they have not come up since then.

Reflection Questions for Readers: How might cultural values and the recent evaluation contribute to this situation? What assumptions might Taylor be making? How can Taylor re-engage with Kyla? If Taylor could go back to before she evaluated Kyla, how might she address some of her concerns in a more culturally engaged manner?

Had Taylor communicated feedback from a place of exploration, this situation may not have come to pass. She could have noticed that what she perceived as a lack of enthusiasm may be due to factors such as emotional display rules that vary across cultures and approached Kyla with a question along the lines of "I'm wondering what you're liking and disliking about working with this population/specialty so far?" to get a sense of Kyla's perceptions. She could have created space to explore some of Kyla's behavior by checking her own assumptions or disclosing her thought process. For example, she could say,

> I'm used to students asking me more questions, which I realize is how I often measure their level of engagement with the work but may not be a fair barometer. I might be misreading how engaged you are given you don't often have questions and your answers to my questions are short. Can you help me understand how engaged in this rotation you feel?

Taylor could also examine her assumption that "enthusiasm" is a prerequisite for the work and what that communicates to students about their place in the profession.

A helpful strategy to assess your feedback to students is a self-audit. Review copies of the evaluations you have given past students with attention to patterns connected to identity or cultural factors. It can be intimidating or anxiety-provoking to hold yourself up to scrutiny, but try to approach this exercise with an open mind. The point is to help identify blind spots and create awareness so you can better address your own biases, not to beat yourself up. Some guilt and embarrassment are normative, as is the instinct to rationalize our behavior or minimize the significance of what we find. Try to notice these sensations without lingering or feeding them, instead focusing on your goal of being a more culturally engaged supervisor. Remind yourself that growth is rarely comfortable, but avoidance of these issues is not acceptable. If you do not have copies of previous evaluations, you may be able to get them from the program(s) with which you have worked. If you are keeping evaluations, make sure you store them in a Family Educational Rights and Privacy Act–compliant manner and that any additional material you create as part of your self-audit is de-identified and protects student confidentiality.

Whether or not your audit identifies patterns, it is important to continue monitoring the feedback you provide. It can be challenging to catch our own biases in real time, so we have developed a list of questions to help you identify warning signs that your intended feedback might be impacted by cultural biases. Pay particular attention to summative or formal feedback (see Chapter 8) because these higher stakes assessments can trigger more severe consequences.

- Do you give this kind of feedback regularly (i.e., about a normative growth area for supervisees)? If not, what specifically is sparking you to give it now?
- Are there certain populations of students who are more likely to receive this type of feedback from you?

- Are there types of feedback you hesitate to provide or feel discomfort in bringing up with students? (See Chapter 7.) What are the origins of that discomfort, and are they tied to identity or cultural values?
- Can you connect the feedback to the student's goals, the Accreditation Council for Genetic Counseling's (2019a) practice-based competencies, assessment questions provided by the student's program, organizational policy, or the NSGC's (2018) code of ethics? If not, what is the basis for the feedback?
- Are you ascribing motive or intention behind behaviors you think need to be corrected? If so, what evidence do you have to support your assessment?

Caution Regarding "Professionalism"

Be very careful any time you feel yourself about to invoke the concept of professionalism when discussing norms or expectations with students. The term "unprofessional" has long been weaponized against individuals who do not identify in the majority to force them to assimilate to the status quo created by dominant identities, especially in domains that have nothing to do with performance of the actual tasks (e.g., hair styles, visible tattoos, and styles of dress). We highly prefer language focused on what is "effective" rather than "professional." "Effective" requires the context of a specific goal or intention related to the practice of genetic counseling as well as consideration of session, patient, clinic, and societal variables. What is effective in one situation may not be effective in another, which introduces space for dialogue, multiple "correct" answers/perspectives, and dynamic nuance. "Professionalism," on the other hand, implies universality. Violations of professionalism raise concerns of whether someone is appropriate for the field and are more likely to trigger shame in a student rather than an opportunity to collaborate on devising a more effective method of achieving the intended outcome. There are certainly issues of professionalism that supervisors need to assess with students (e.g., returning phone calls from patients, being prepared for appointments, and following ethical mandates), but we need to make sure that when using this term, we are correctly tying it to something critical to the function of a genetic counselor.

Communication of Culture

The supervisory relationship, a tenet of the REM-S, forms the working alliance (see Chapter 1). This relationship is built through sharing of experiences that shape the supervision process and relationship, including personal characteristics and attitudes (Wherley et al., 2015). As discussed previously, however, Dewey et al. (2022) found cultural factors, specifically race/ethnicity, were not often discussed in the building of genetic counseling supervisory relationships. As supervisors in their study noted, for example, "I think it's just a dialogue [about race/ethnicity] that doesn't happen, so that's why it's hard for me to figure out exactly what I'm trying to say, because it's something we don't talk about a lot" (White participant, p. 5) and "They're [students] pretty much all the same [race/ethnicity], so I've treated them all the same. I can't really compare and contrast" (non-White participant, p. 6).

There are many possible reasons these conversations do not occur—limited time, prioritization of client-centered education, discomfort, and a desire to treat all students equally (Dewey et al., 2022). Lack of communication may have considerable effects on the student, supervisor, supervision relationship, and genetic counseling services. Consider this scenario:

Scenario 4

Nina is a White-passing student who identifies as Latina. She just started a cardiogenetics rotation. Nina is observing her supervisor counsel a Latine couple whose daughter was recently diagnosed with a heart arrhythmia concerning for long QT syndrome. The parents continually look to Nina as her supervisor counsels them about the genetics of long QT. When the supervisor steps out of the room, the couple begins to talk to Nina openly about their confusion and distress over this overwhelming diagnostic process. At some point, Nina begins to speak in Spanish with the couple and learns more about the couple's social situation and lack of understanding of support in the face of their daughter's health concerns. When the supervisor returns to the room, the conversation immediately halts. The supervisor continued the session but after, in debriefing with Nina, the supervisor remarked, "I didn't even know you spoke a different language!"

It appears there were missed opportunities to communicate and share cultural similarities and differences for Nina and her supervisor.

Reflection Questions for Readers: As Nina's supervisor, what would your thoughts and feelings have been walking back into the room and hearing Nina speaking fluently with the couple? How do you think Nina felt when her supervisor commented on her Spanish proficiency? How could Nina's supervisor have begun to discuss Nina's cultural background earlier? How did Nina's cultural identities create different opportunities for her with this couple? How could those be opportunities for future sessions?

Given her Latina background and Spanish proficiency, Nina brings invaluable experiences and perspectives to her rotations and the genetic counseling profession (de Leon et al., 2022). Assumptions, however, based on Nina's White-passing appearance, likely did not prompt her supervisor to ask more about the background she brings to genetic counseling. This could have been an unfortunate missed opportunity for both Nina and her supervisor. Perhaps Nina felt relief at being able to speak in Spanish with this couple and potentially begin to counsel more authentically. It is hoped that her supervisor can debrief this session and begin culture sharing in a way that is safe, mutual, and responsive.

This scenario and the previous ones highlight another important aspect. Given the power imbalance in supervision, students are unlikely to initiate discussions of culture. Cultural broaching is a "counselor's [supervisor's] invitation to examine the role of race, ethnicity, and other cultural factors within the counseling [supervision] process" (Day-Vines et al., 2018, cited in King, 2019, p. 87). The supervisor is responsible for an ongoing process of inviting students to examine culture within the supervision relationship. Communication about culture is part of building the supervisory relationship and is fostered by an environment of trust and support. Not discussing culture can invalidate important components of students' identities. A colorblind approach to supervision minimizes the importance of culture, and when negative experiences arise (e.g., racism and microaggression), supervisees may feel little permission for or recognition of its significance (Neville et al., 2006). This can be especially imperative if the supervisor belongs to a dominant cultural group, which adds to the already existing power differential. King (2019) stresses the importance of timing in broaching, as well as the careful use of language.

Within a strong working alliance, culture sharing can create a time for supervisors and students to understand their shared and different experiences and ways they impact their relationship and genetic counseling work. Constantine's (1997) questions offer several suggested prompts for culture sharing in supervision. Appendix 4C contains a structure to begin culture sharing with students based on Constantine's questions. The structure includes setting ground rules and scheduling time to discuss the questions.

Challenging Issues: Microaggression/Racism

Cultural conversations in supervision often begin in relationship to students' work with clients (Dewey et al., 2022). Often, these conversations can turn to educational components (e.g., How can language be clear?) or working with translators, rather than discussing the interpersonal dynamics and interactions that can occur when cultural differences are apparent between the student and the client. For students from underrepresented backgrounds, this can bring both opportunities and challenges depending on shared backgrounds with clients (Carmichael et al., 2021). When students experience challenges with clients, specifically in the form of microaggression ("daily verbal, behavioral or environmental slights, whether intentional or unintentional, that communicate hostile, derogatory, or negative attitudes toward stigmatized or culturally marginalized groups" [Sue, 2010, p. xvi]) and racist comments, supervisors have a critical role in addressing them. Consider this scenario:

Scenario 5

Diana is a genetic counseling student just weeks from graduation, and she has worked fairly independently with patients during her final pediatric rotation. Diana identifies as Asian Indian, and although proficient in English, she does speak with a slight accent. From the start of the session (even during interaction in the waiting room), Julie, her supervisor, noticed the child's parents seemed uneasy with Diana. They made little eye contact and kept looking to Julie when responding to Diana's questions. At one point, the father started to roll his eyes and interrupted Diana. He said, "Excuse me, I don't know why you need to ask all of these questions, and we can hardly understand you. We'd like to work with her [looking at Julie]." Diana looked at Julie helplessly, and Julie stepped in to finish the session.

Although potentially uncomfortable, how can supervisors navigate these situations for students with clients?

Reflection Questions for Readers: How would you have felt as Julie in observing the parents' behaviors? What emotions and thoughts are you noticing for yourself? Although jumping in to finish the session may have eased the immediate tension, what do you think was the impact on Diana? On Julie? If you were Julie, what would be your next steps after this session?

As Diana's supervisor, you have begun to sense the parents' unease with Diana early in the session. Would that have been a time to anticipate the need to address what is unfolding and the potential for a negative treatment of Diana? During the session, Julie likely did her best to quickly resolve the tension in the room and, quite frankly, get the session over with. Yet, it ignored what transpired during the session—a racist statement toward Diana. In that moment, Julie may not have known how to best help Diana. At minimum, offering support and resources to Diana through a debrief after the session and at a later time are needed. Moving forward, Julie may have wanted to begin to anticipate these incidents in a more responsive (versus reactive) way and help students anticipate them by discussing with Diana and other students how she can support them in a variety of scenarios—from a resistant to a racist client.

Scenarios such as this one are not uncommon. Microaggressions and racism have been reported by genetic counseling students (Carmichael et al., 2020). These harmful remarks can be experienced from clients, such as the case for Diana, but also from other health care team members and supervisors. Supervisors need to be prepared to address and respond to microaggressions and racist remarks because supervisees are often not in a power position to respond and may be experiencing confusion and hurt based on the comments.

At this point in the supervisory relationship, it is hoped that you have begun to acknowledge and explore with students their cultural identities. In doing so, and by sharing your own, there is a level of trust, vulnerability, and safety that contributes to discussion of cultural concerns and negative experience. Anticipate with the student if and how microaggressions and racist remarks come up in their fieldwork experience and express your desire to address those incidents and be an ally to them. In addition to offering your own perspective and approach to addressing these negative interactions, ask the student how they would like to be supported. This discussion creates a potential action plan, and it also sends a powerful message about the culture of inclusion you hope to create during their rotation.

Sotto-Santiago et al. (2020) suggest the OWTFD approach to responding to racism, discrimination, and microaggressions. Box 4.2 details the approach.

For Scenario 5, OWTFD gives Julie words to help interrupt and respond in the moment to microaggressions:

O: "I noticed you seem uncomfortable" [to the patient's parents as you observe their unease].

W: "Can you tell me what is difficult for you?"

T: "I think we are *all* focusing on what is best for your child."

F: "I feel uncomfortable with what you have just said as I know Diana is a very capable intern."

D: "We are here to help you as a team. We do not change providers because of their identities. I would like for Diana to have the opportunity to help you and your child."

BOX 4.2 The OWTFD Approach to Racism, Discrimination, and Microaggressions

Observe: Provide concrete, factual observations that are not evaluative.
"*I noticed . . .*"
What did you mean?
Think: Thoughts based on observation.
"*I think . . .*"
Feel: Name an emotion so you can take ownership of what you feel instead of the other individual.
"*I feel . . .*"
Desire: A specific request or inquiry about a desired outcome.
"*I would like . . .*"

Source: Sotto-Santiago, S., Mac, J., Duncan, F., & Smith, J. (2020). "I didn't know what to say": Responding to racism, discrimination, and microaggressions with the OWTFD approach. *MedEdPORTAL, 16*, 10971.

Although OWTFD offers guidelines in advocating for students in instances of racism, discrimination, and microaggressions, it is important to consider a couple of caveats when "confronting" a patient. First, patients have the right to decline to be seen or observed by a student. Therefore, before responding within the OWTFD framework, Julie needs to thoughtfully assess whether the parents' resistance to working with Diana is about their desire to not work with any student or if it is about working with *this* student. If the former is suspected, Diana may be asked to observe or not be part of this session because competent patient care is a priority. Second, Julie will want to consult with her supervisor and/or clinic manager about this patient interaction to ensure that her response aligns with institutional polices. There is understandable tension between advocating for appropriate patient care and providing culturally supportive supervision for your student. If institutional policies or guidelines do not exist on addressing and responding to patient racism or discrimination, consider voicing the need for these to be developed and assist in writing and training within your institution.

Finally, always debrief with students after incidents of racism, discrimination, and microaggression. Check in with the student, acknowledge the event directly, and offer support. Ask the student again how you can be helpful to them. Identify resources for them. They may wish to make their graduate program or faculty aware of the incident so they can serve as another support network. The graduate program can also assist you in identifying resources within the program/university system. It is also important to note the toll these situations take on supervisors. They are disturbing and personally and professionally upsetting to witness. Take care of yourself by debriefing and consulting with a trusted colleague.

Continuing the Work

Throughout this chapter, we provided scenarios to illustrate how issues between students and supervisors may manifest and guided you toward salient aspects to consider through the reflection questions for readers. These are important initial steps, but to continue building self-efficacy in engaging culturally with students, you need lived experience having these conversations. What seems straightforward on paper can become tricky when we vocalize with others and consider the nonverbal messages we are also sending. We recommend starting with simulated situations (e.g., see Learning Activity 4.4).

As discussed previously, we chose to focus our examples primarily around race and ethnicity, but culturally engaged supervision requires attention to the full range of cultural identities. The strategies we have shared can be applied to other aspects of culture, and to aid you in making this transition, we created additional scenarios related to gender, disability, and religion (see Learning Activity 4.5). Use these as a launching point to continue expanding the range of culture-related topics with which you engage.

Closing Thoughts

In this chapter, we briefly summarized important terminology and background to set the foundation for culturally engaged supervision. As relationship-focused supervisors, we foreground the importance of creating space for conversations about JEDI issues as central to this work. Digging into these topics with students may lead to uncomfortable moments but will unlock the possibility for deeper connections that support the next generation of genetic counselors in being authentic in their identities and feeling valued as members of the community. By suggesting some entry points to these conversations and strategies for developing self-awareness, we hope to have helped you take a step in the ongoing journey toward culturally engaged supervision practice. Sustained engagement is the only way to enact real change.

Learning Activities

Most learning activities can be adapted for dyad or small group discussions or for written exercises. Time estimates are provided for discussions, but additional time should be allotted for large group processing.

Activity 4.1 Cultural Self-Awareness

Complete the worksheet contained in Appendix 4A based on P. Hays' (1996) ADDRESSING model to help you understand your intersectional identity. With a partner or in a small group, discuss the following questions about your responses to each column:

Column 1
- What identities were easy to name? What were difficult?
- What do you notice about your identities? Are they dominant or marginalized identities? Both? Neither?
- How does this change in the various contexts in which you live your life (e.g., work, friend groups, and family)?

Column 2
- How do these identities present opportunities in supervision? Challenges?
- What biases and assumptions do you bring to supervision based on these identities?
- What are ways that you manage these biases and assumptions?

Column 3
- How do similarities in identifies between you and your supervisees impact your supervision? Differences?
- In what ways do your expectations about similarities and differences influence how you may want to approach discussing culture with your supervisees?

Column 4

- For the identities you wish to share, begin to think about how you may comfortably share this with your supervisee.
- For the identities you do not wish to share, take time to reflect on how these are private for you. What boundaries do you set to maintain your own sense of safety and privacy in supervision?

Share your worksheets with a partner or in small groups.

Estimated time: 45-60 minutes

Activity 4.2 Communication Style Dimensions

Complete the communication style worksheet contained in Appendix 4B. Then share your responses with a partner. As part of the discussion, reflect on the advantages and challenges of where you are on each dimension.

Estimated time: 30 minutes

Activity 4.3 Culture Sharing in Supervision: Dyad Role Plays

With a partner, take turns playing the role of supervisor and student who are at the beginning of their supervision relationship. Using portions of the Culture Sharing Worksheet contained in Appendix 4C, identify two or three ground rules (see Step 1), and then discuss two of the questions listed in Step 2 (the "supervisor" can select one question and the "student" can select one question). Finally, discuss what it was like to engage in this process.

Estimated time: 30 minutes

Activity 4.4 Challenging Situations: Dyad Role Plays

Using Scenarios 2–5 from this chapter, re-enact each scenario as a role play with a partner. We encourage you to take some risks and try things that may be outside your comfort zone as you role play. This is an excellent opportunity to get feedback from peers.

For each role play scenario, we recommend the following process:

1. Assign yourself to be either the supervisor or the student. It can be helpful to have an observer as well. The observer can write down specific phrases that either worked well or need to be refined.

2. Although the most important part to role play might be the moment immediately after the scenario takes place, play out what led up to the scenario itself to simulate some of the emotional energy that might be present in the room. For example, in Scenario 5, having someone play the parent will bring stronger reactions into the role play.

3. Use the strategies in the chapter and your answers to the *Reflection Questions for Readers* to guide how you engage with the student.

4. Many scenarios include a rupture in the relationship between the supervisor and the student. What would be your short- and long-term strategies to repair this rupture?

5. Reflect on your experience with your role-play partner (and observers, if applicable). Take notes on their feedback as well as your reflections on the experience.

6. Repeat the role play from the other perspective. This gives your partner a chance to try their own approach to the scenario and gives you lived experience in the role of a student. *Pay attention to your emotional reactions, but remember that depending on your identities, you may have quite different responses to words and behaviors compared to your students.*

7. You might want to repeat the role play several times with different emotional undertones (from the perspective of the student and supervisor) to practice a variety of responses.

8. Use these suggested reflection questions to debrief following your role plays:
   - What were your feelings and thoughts in the role of the supervisor? As the student?
   - As the supervisor:
     - What did you like about your approach?
     - What would you have done differently?
   - As the student:
     - What did you like about the supervisor's approach?
     - What would you like to have been done differently?
   - What was unexpected or surprising that occurred in doing this role play?
   - How will this role play change your supervision moving forward?

Estimated time: 30 minutes per scenario and discussion

Note: Ideally, you would record the role play so you could watch it later and critique your performance. If you do record, make sure everyone is aware of the recording ahead of time and there are agreements in place about how the recording will be used, who will have access to it, and how long it will be retained. Watching ourselves is often uncomfortable, but it provides excellent insights about our nonverbal communication and allows for more careful review of the nuanced language used throughout the exercise.

Activity 4.5 Culturally Engaged Supervision

Part I: Discussion

In small groups, engage in a discussion of each of the scenarios listed below. Use the following self-reflection process to guide discussion of each scenario:

Cultural self-awareness: Use these questions from the ADDRESSING framework worksheet in Appendix 4A.

- As the supervisor, how do *your* identities align or differ from those of the student?
- How do these similarities or differences influence biases and assumptions you bring to this situation?
- How do you anticipate growth in cultural self-awareness may assist your work with this student?

Communication of expectations

- What can you infer about the communication expectations between the supervisor and the student in this scenario?
- What are some potential cultural explanations/hypotheses for the similarities and differences in communication style?
- As the supervisor, how would you broach a conversation about communication expectations with this student?

Communication of feedback

- Moving forward, how can you re-engage with this student in a more culturally aware and sensitive manner?
- How will you incorporate this student's cultural identity into your feedback?

Communication of culture

- How can you begin to discuss this student's cultural identity and background earlier in the supervision relationship?
- What of your own cultural identities will you share with this student and how?

Addressing microaggression and racism

- How can/could you anticipate and plan for experiences of microaggression and/or racism with this student?
- What are some ways you can be an ally to this student during an incident of microaggression and/or racism? After the incident?
- What microaggressions might you yourself commit with this student, and how can you attempt to repair ruptures to the supervisory working alliance?

Estimated time: 45 minutes

Note: Part I can be a written exercise.

Scenario

Parker is a nonbinary student who uses they/them pronouns and whose gender expression is male. They are currently rotating with Kristen in a laboratory setting and work in a remote capacity with most communications and clients seen via phone, email, and video. For the past couple of weeks, Kristen notices that in large group laboratory meetings, her colleagues often misgender Parker. Although uncomfortable, she understands why this could happen and, in fact, she has been guilty of the same thing. In a recent video conference, Parker was referred to as "he," and Kristen watched their expression change from engaged to deflated on the video call. Kristen schedules a meeting with Parker to check in but is feeling uncertain about what to do and does not want to make assumptions about Parker's reactions.

Scenario

Jennifer is rotating with Max in the cancer genetics clinic. Prior to her rotation, Jennifer's program director contacted Max to share that Jennifer may need accommodations because of a visual impairment. She told Max, "I wouldn't worry about it too much as Jennifer is an excellent student and so you won't even notice!" In working with Jennifer for the past couple of weeks, Max has begun to agree with the program director that Jennifer is excellent—well-prepared, great with patients, and very knowledgeable. Today, Max was observing Jennifer counsel a patient who had done direct-to-consumer genetic testing and had an "abnormal" result. The patient handed Jennifer the test results during the session, and it became clear that Jennifer was having difficulty reading and, in turn, interpreting the result. The patient seemed to be getting impatient as Jennifer took a long time reading. To avoid a potential confrontation, Max took over the session and counseled the patient. After the session, Max told Jennifer they would talk more about this case later.

Scenario

Susan is 2 weeks into her rotation in a prenatal clinic with Kelly. She identifies as a conservative Christian. She was nervous to start this rotation because she knew her religious beliefs inform her personal objections to abortion. On the first day of the rotation, she told Kelly that conversations about termination make her uncomfortable, but she knew part of her role as a genetic counselor is presenting all options to patients. Susan observed for the first week and took family histories the second week. This afternoon is the first day Susan is going to discuss termination in session. Tamara and Winston are devastated after a 20-week ultrasound noted major abnormalities. Susan did a great job presenting the options available to the couple, after which Tamara looked her in the eye and asked, "What would you do if you were me?" Susan quickly replied, "Well I could never choose abortion because of my strong Christian values, but you're the only one who can make this decision for your pregnancy." Tamara leaned over, looked at the floor, and started to cry. Winston scowled and started to rub his partner's back. At this point, Kelly noticed the crucifix necklace Tamara was wearing and took over the session. The afternoon was full of back-to-back sessions, but Kelly noticed Susan seemed less engaged than normal. It is now the end of the day when Susan and Kelly are scheduled to debrief about the afternoon's patients.

Part II: Role Plays

Take turns as supervisor, student, and observer for the scenarios described in Part I. After each role play, the observer and student give feedback to the supervisor about how they addressed the issue.

Estimated time: 30–45 minutes

Appendix 4A
Cultural Identities and Their Intersection

ADDRESSING Component	List your identities	How do these identities influence your supervision?	Check which identities you expect students to share with you	Check which identities you feel are important to share with students
Age and generational influences				
Developmental disabilities				
Disabilities acquired later in life				
Religion and spiritual orientation				
Ethnic and racial identity				
Socioeconomic status				
Sexual orientation				
Indigenous heritage				
National origin				
Gender				
Other *What other identities are important to you?*				

Adapted from Hays, P. (2008). *Addressing cultural complexities in practice: Assessment, diagnosis, and therapy* (2nd ed.). American Psychological Association.

Appendix 4B
Communication Style Dimensions

The purpose of this worksheet is to identify how you tend to communicate to help you understand how you may come across and identify areas in which conflict or miscommunication might occur. Rate yourself on each of the following dimensions. Try not to overthink; rather, go with your first instinct. Try to answer according to how you communicate when in your supervisor or supervisee role. For example, in your personal life, you might use a lot of analogies, but that may not be the case in supervision.

There are no right or wrong answers. There are advantages and challenges to each end of the spectrum.

Low Context			**High Context**
Communication is explicit, direct, and works equally well in writing and orally			Communication is indirect, relies on body language/tone for understanding, and works better in person
Task-Focused			**Relationship-Focused**
Tend to connect directly to what needs to be done first; relationship develops as tasks are completed			Tend to focus on interpersonal dynamics first; productivity develops as harmony emerges
Internal Processing			**External Processing**
Prefer to stop and think quietly before responding			Talking helps clarify my ideas

Literal	Symbolic
Tend to use technical details to explain concepts	Tend to use metaphors or analogies to explain concepts
Collaborative	**Hierarchical**
Expect to come up with solutions together and equally value everyone's contributions	Expect to have my instructions followed without having to explain myself
Empirical	**Instinctual**
Tend to wait to have evidence before speaking up; like structure	Tend to trust intuition and follow hunches in conversation; like flexibility
Low Disclosure	**High Disclosure**
Tend to hold back personal thoughts and experiences; maintain stricter boundaries	Quickly and easily share examples from my own life and experiences

What role does silence play in my communication? (When I'm silent, it likely means . . .

Note. This worksheet is not intended to definitively classify your communication style but, rather, to stimulate conversation between you and your student. You may also find it useful to have your colleagues complete the worksheet based on their perceptions of you, as their perspectives may help you anticipate how your students might see you.

Appendix 4C
Culture Sharing Worksheet

This worksheet comprises a suggested structure to begin discussing cultural identities in supervision.

Step 1: Begin by sharing with the student your desire to understand more about the experiences they bring to supervision and to their fieldwork rotation. Also state that you would like to share a bit more about yourself as this will help them understand you and the background you bring to supervision. Discuss the student's comfort with this process and let them know that you would first like to set these ground rules:

Ground Rules

The following are some suggested ground rules, along with blank space for adding ground rules that you and your student identify:

- *This is a safe and confidential space.* You will not be forced to share what you do not feel comfortable disclosing. I will respect your confidentiality and not share what you disclose with others. I ask you to do the same about what I share.
- *Culture is important and valued.* I believe culture is important in understanding each other. I will not judge but, rather, value the cultural backgrounds you bring to supervision.
- *Culture sharing is an ongoing process.* This is not a one-time discussion. We will continue to discuss how our cultural identities inform our supervision relationship and genetic counseling work.
- [Fill in]

- [Fill in]
- [Fill in]

Give the student a copy of the ground rules.

Step 2: Give the student a copy of the following questions to review and schedule a time in supervision to begin discussing them. Determine with the student which questions to start with. We recognize the time for these discussions may be limited, and thus we bolded questions that may be most relevant in genetic counseling.
Constantine's (1997) questions:

1. **What are the main demographic variables (e.g., race/ethnicity, gender, sexual orientation, age, socioeconomic status, spiritual tradition, etc.) that make up my cultural identities?**
2. What worldviews (e.g., assumptions, biases, values, etc.) do I bring to the supervision relationship based on these cultural identities?
3. What value systems, based on my demographic identities, are inherent in the way I approach supervision?
4. What value systems, based on my demographic identities, underlie the strategies and techniques I use (or, if a student, prefer) in supervision?
5. What knowledge do I possess about the worldviews of supervisors/students who have different cultural identities from me?
6. **What skills do I possess for working with supervisors/students who have different cultural identities from me?**
7. **What are some of my struggles and challenges in working with supervisors/students who are culturally different from me?**
8. **How do I address or resolve these issues?**
9. In what ways would I like to improve my abilities in working with culturally diverse supervisors/students?

Step 3: Discuss your responses. Be realistic about what questions you will be able to discuss and set aside adequate and uninterrupted time to do so privately. We recommend discussing one or two questions at a time. Schedule future times to discuss additional questions.

Step 4. At the end of each discussion, debrief. Talk about what it was like to engage in this discussion, how to use this information to improve your supervision work together, and how to use it to inform your work with clients.

*Adapted from Constantine, M. G. (1997). Facilitating multicultural competency in counseling supervision: Operationalizing a practical framework. In D. B. Pope-Davis & H. L. K. Coleman (Eds.), *Multicultural counseling competencies* (pp. 310–324). Sage.

Models of Supervisor and Student Development

PATRICIA MCCARTHY VEACH

Objectives

- Describe models of supervisor and student development.
- Identify characteristics associated with novice versus more advanced supervisors and students.
- Describe strategies for promoting supervisor and student development.
- Identify characteristics and behaviors indicating student readiness for counseling independently.
- Describe strategies for facilitating student transition to counseling independently.

An expert is someone who has succeeded in making decisions and judgements simpler through knowing what to pay attention to and what to ignore.
—EDWARD DE BONO (AS CITED IN BRAINY QUOTE, N.D.-B)

Supervisor and Supervisee Developmental Models

When you hear the terms *novice* and *advanced* to describe supervisors, what comes to mind? What about when you hear the terms *novice* and *advanced* students? Do you notice any similarities in your images of novice supervisors and students? Are there any similarities in your images of advanced supervisors and students?

Developmental models describe progressive stages of supervisor and supervisee development and discrete characteristics and skills associated with each stage (Behavioral Health Providers Association of New Mexico, n.d.). The following sections contain descriptions of several models. You will notice similar themes in supervisor and supervisee developmental processes and outcomes.

Supervisor Models

Supervisor development models are largely adaptations of mental health counselor development models. Of the few existing models, all include three or four stages of development. Each model emphasizes shifts in professional identity and skills that occur with experience and training, and all but one (Alonso's model; Alonso, 1983) describe a relatively short-term process. Three sets of factors influence development: self-identity, the supervision relationship, and the administrative structure of the work setting (e.g., opportunity or lack thereof for peer supervision/consultation). Every model depicts ultimate developmental outcomes as positive. As primarily described by Bernard and Goodyear (2014, pp. 290–293), there are five models:

> *Alonso model* (Alonso, 1983): This three-stage model has both a psychodynamic and a developmental basis and reflects a supervisor's entire career.
> *Novice stage*—This stage is characterized by developing a self-identity as a supervisor and coping with anxiety over being a novice (especially when supervisees are close in age and/or experience to the supervisor).
> *Midcareer stage*—Supervisors are moving toward being an ideal mentor as their focus shifts from themselves to others.

Late career stage—This stage reflects supervisors' ability to maintain self-esteem about their supervision skills if they practice in a Western culture in which older people are sometimes devalued. To the extent that they overcome devaluation attempts, supervisors achieve the status of "village elder," appreciated for their knowledge, skills, and wisdom.

Hess model (Hess, 1986, 1987): This model has three stages.

Beginning stage—The transition from being a student to a supervisor often produces role ambiguity, uncertainty about supervision techniques, self-consciousness, and sensitivity to criticism from supervisees and other colleagues. Many supervisors initially compensate by being overly structured, focus primarily on the supervisee's clients, and they use teaching techniques (likely directive rather than evocative ones; see Chapter 2).

Exploration stage—This stage is characterized by increased competence and confidence in one's role and performance as a supervisor and a growing belief in the value of supervision. Supervisors at this stage are likely to slip into one of two response sets: being too restrictive in their roles or being too intrusive with supervisees (e.g., delving into issues unrelated to clinical work). Either response set may create conflict and lead to supervisee resistance.

Confirmation of supervisor identity stage—At this stage, supervisors have a strong professional identity, feel gratified by their supervision work, and are proud of their supervisees' successes. They are less likely to rely on others for validation of their capabilities as supervisors, and they relate not only at a cognitive level to their supervisees' needs but also from an emotional/relational perspective.

Rodenhauser model (Rodenhauser, 1994, 1997): There are four stages.

Emulation stage—New supervisors try to be like their previous supervisor role models. They gradually recognize imitation is insufficient and begin to move away from overidentifying with their former supervisors.

Conceptualization stage—Supervisors in this stage search for methods, guidelines, and processes to define their approach to supervision. Discussion with peers is a commonly used resource in this process.

Incorporation stage—At this stage, supervisors are becoming more aware of the centrality of the supervisory relationship to supervision processes and outcomes. They are more attuned to the effects of their interpersonal style on the supervisee and their work. They are more aware of individual and cultural differences and how they may affect supervision and supervisee service provision.

Consolidation stage—Supervisors are integrating knowledge and experience into their approach to supervision. Particularly noteworthy, they can recognize and address supervisees' countertransference about supervision without being overly intrusive.

Stoltenberg and McNeill's (2011) integrated developmental model: This model assumes supervisors and supervisees transition through four similar stages. Stoltenberg and McNeill describe supervisor levels as follows:

Level I—Supervisors are anxious and eager to do the *right thing*. They are often mechanical and structured in their interactions, act as if they are *the expert*, and insist supervisees perform exactly as directed (e.g., a supervisor who requires a moderately advanced genetic counseling student to memorize and use exact wording when providing counseling services to clients). A Level I approach may sometimes be effective with beginning students who are eager for structure, but it may "fail" with more advanced students, leading to conflict, resistance, and loss of self-confidence.

Level II—Supervisors are prone to confusion and conflict as they recognize the complexity of supervision. They may fluctuate in their motivation to be in this role and blame their supervisees for difficulties being a supervisor. Fortunately, Stoltenberg and McNeill believe Level II is a short-lived stage.

Level III—Individuals have a stable level of motivation toward being supervisors. They function with autonomy and are honest and more accurate in their self-evaluations.

Level IV—Individuals at this stage are *master supervisors*. They can work effectively with supervisees at all developmental levels and usually do not prefer supervising individuals at a particular level.

Watkins' Supervisor Complexity Model (Watkins, 1993): This is a four-stage model.

Role shock—Supervisors at this level feel like an imposter and experience conflict over "playing the role" of supervisor. They respond to their feelings by taking a very concrete, rule-oriented approach (e.g., spending inordinate amounts of supervision time correcting and discussing a student's follow-up letters to clients). Novice supervisors may adopt a self-protective stance, withdrawing from supervisees or imposing a too-rigid structure.

Role recovery and transition—Supervisors at this stage are beginning to develop a supervisor identity, have more self-confidence, and are better able to realistically assess their strengths and limitations, although their nascent self-assessments fluctuate quite a bit. They are also growing in their ability to manage ambiguity and to recognize supervision dynamics such as transference and countertransference, but they may not be as skilled at addressing them.

Role consolidation—Supervisors at this stage are continuing to grow into the supervisor role. They are more consistent in how they think about and approach supervision, gain further self-confidence, and shift to a more supportive rather than a controlling/directive stance with supervisees. They are better able to address transference and countertransference.

Role mastery—Supervisors have a solid foundation with respect to their self-concept and a well-developed supervisor identity. Their supervisory approach is well-integrated, consistent, and individualized.

Common Themes in Supervisor Models

Supervisor models suggest a general process involving transition to an integrated identity. With positive development comes less anxiety, greater flexibility, increased confidence, self-awareness, and authenticity; greater focus on the supervisee in the form of support, encouragement, and guidance, and recognition of the role of supervisor in those processes; more attention to dynamics such as transference and countertransference; and greater awareness of the influence of individual traits and cultural factors on supervision. The distinctions between supervisors at various levels of development, however, are not always obvious. Watkins (2012) notes, "The models seemingly have their clearest, most identifiable distinctions at the beginning and end points; it is the middle parts that become a bit more fuzzy and difficult to track" (p. 70).

Missing in these models is discussion of why some supervisors fail to develop and/or deteriorate in their supervision work. Research suggests experience alone does not lead to increased supervision skills; it must be accompanied by training and ongoing self-reflection (Watkins, 2012). A desire to improve, openness to self-examination, and willingness to try new approaches "seem to be both the prerequisites and lubricant for the initiation and maintenance of any sort of supervisor development process" (Watkins, 2012, p. 71). It is also likely that other professional experiences, such as compassion fatigue, burnout, and lack of institutional support for supervision (e.g., reduced caseload, peer supervision/consultation), have deleterious effects on supervisor development.

Supervisee Developmental Models

"I feel like a fraud, the [supervisee] said. "You are," answered the . . . supervisor. . . . "We all begin as frauds. . . . That is the nature of the learning. . . . As we read, apply theories and techniques, and learn the vicissitudes of the patient–[practitioner]–supervisor interaction, we grow to be less and less fraudulent, and eventually mature into the real thing."

—WATKINS (2012, P. 46)

One of the most widely cited supervisee developmental models is the four-stage integrated development model (IDM) (Stoltenberg et al., 1998; Stoltenberg & McNeill, 2011). As mentioned previously, the IDM assumes similar developmental paths for supervisors and supervisees. The stages of the supervisee model (Behavioral Health Providers Association of New Mexico, n.d.; Bernard & Goodyear, 2014) are as follows:

> *Level 1*—At this stage, supervisees are novices who have limited training and/or experience. They are simultaneously highly motivated to learn but anxious about their ability to do so and about being evaluated. They are interested in learning "the right way" to do things, need structure, are dependent on their supervisor, self-focused rather than client-focused, and limited in their ability to self-evaluate accurately (e.g., some novice supervisees may be overly confident [Venne & Coleman, 2010]).
>
> *Level 2*—At this mid-level stage, supervisees begin moving toward greater autonomy, realistically based confidence, and a focus on clients. Movement in these directions can be like a roller coaster, however, with wide fluctuations. Instability often relates to how well (or not) the last client session went.
>
> *Level 3*—Supervisees at this stage are working to develop their own counseling style, they are more stable in their

self-confidence, and they are better able to be both client- and self-focused and to use these foci in the best interests of the client.

Level 3i (integrated)—This is a consolidation stage in which supervisees have merged their knowledge, skills, and experiences into a personal style that would allow them to function across all types of practice specialties and skill domains. At this stage, they have an accurate sense of their strengths and growth areas.

Table 5.1 contains characteristics of novice versus advanced student supervisees as I have experienced them and as described in the literature. I regard each characteristic as a continuum.

Supervisor and Supervisee Developmental Challenges: Parallel Processes

Development requires intense practice—"a long obedience in the same direction."

—KARON (2017)

Both supervisor and supervisee models imply that development occurs linearly, but that is not the case. Individuals can be more advanced in some respects (e.g., highly attuned empathically to student and/or client needs) and less advanced in others (e.g., lacking in self-confidence), and they can sometimes appear to regress in their development. Thus, they may be in different stages simultaneously. Regarding more advanced student supervisees, it is important to avoid assuming they have had certain prior experiences. Sometimes there are "holes" in their training opportunities and thus the corresponding skills may not be as developed as you would expect. For instance, a student who has been unable to participate in positive test results sessions will be anxious when leading such a session at your site and possibly more awkward in their approach.

TABLE 5.1 Novice Versus Advanced Student Characteristics

Characteristic	Novice Student	Advanced Student
Dependence	Highly dependent on client and supervisor feedback.	Better able to self-evaluate accurately. Note that an advanced student who is dependent may be experiencing countertransference but be unable to recognize it as such without the aid of a supervisor.
Autonomy	Looks to the supervisor for direction.	More self-directed.
Confidence	Either less confident or overly confident.	More confident, and their confidence is based on realistic self-appraisal.
Anxiety	Experiences more global anxiety about their competencies.	Has more skill-specific anxiety. May have more performance anxiety, believing they must appear "expert."
Flexibility	More rigid; rule-bound; secretly wishes there was an instruction manual. Feels safer emphasizing *genetics* over *feelings* and following a prepared outline no matter what is going on in a session.	More flexible/fluid in their counseling. More comfortable tackling psychosocial issues. Better able to adjust their agenda to be responsive to what is going on in a session.

(continued)

TABLE 5.1 (Continued)

Characteristic	Novice Student	Advanced Student
Motivation for supervision	Scared about, but also eager for, supervision. Often feel as if they can't get enough.	May also fear supervision (especially if they had a prior negative experience); may regard supervision as a burden in a busy schedule; may welcome feedback, especially on self-directed goals.
Personal responsibility	Either feels overly responsible for everything that happens in a genetic counseling session or seems oblivious to their impact.	Has a more realistic and balanced perspective of their role and responsibility. Can more accurately appraise their impact.
Self-concept	Has a fragile, not well-defined self-concept—has many questions about their professional identity (What is my role? What am I supposed to be doing?), their strengths and limitations, and their effectiveness. Self-concept shifts fairly easily due to others' reactions.	Has a more stable and clear self-concept and is more resistant to fluctuations due to specific client and/or supervisor reactions.

TABLE 5.1 (Continued)

Characteristic	Novice Student	Advanced Student
Supervision needs	*Somewhat* more homogeneous with respect to having a high need for support and guidance.	More heterogeneous in their needs due to unique prior rotation experiences and the extent to which their skills have developed.
Supervision goals	Has less clear, precise, and/or unrealistic goals. Often has glamorized expectations.	Has more specific, realistic, personalized goals and more reasonable expectations. Note that some advanced students (e.g., those in a final rotation) may inaccurately perceive they have little left to learn.

The developmental process is not easy for either supervisors or supervisees because it simultaneously involves cognitive, affective, and behavioral changes sparked by the many challenges encountered throughout one's professional activities (Falender & Shafranske, 2021; Watkins, 2012). And the developmental process never ends. I like to remind supervisors and students that there are no terminal skill levels when it comes to supervision and genetic counseling skills.

Models of novice supervisee and supervisor development suggest novices face similar developmental challenges they must work through in order to progress. Box 5.1 describes these challenges.

BOX 5.1 Typical Supervisee and Supervisor Developmental Challenges

Lack of a clear sense of one's role—"What am I supposed to be doing?"

Lack of confidence—Self-doubt leads to supervisees being dependent on supervisors and clients for validation, while supervisors are dependent on supervisees and/or colleagues for validation.

Anxiety—Fear of being deficient regarding one or more competencies; worried about being evaluated.

Rigidity—"If I follow certain rules, I won't lose control and things will turn out ok."

Feeling threatened by dynamics—Wanting to stick to content and avoid emotions; "misses/misunderstands" transference and countertransference dynamics.

Lack of focus/direction—Have little or no theoretical model and/or prior experience to guide service provision, which can lead to a laissez-faire approach: "Since I don't know what I'm doing, I'll wing it."

Using time inefficiently—Every encounter requires a great deal of effort, energy, and time, which may interfere with other responsibilities and reduce overall efficiency.

Lacking a comparative base—Every counseling or supervising interaction is additive given the lack of prior "normative" experiences. Although additive experiences are valuable, lack of a base means the individual is unable to discern with relative confidence what substandard, average, and superior performance look like.

Questioning one's credibility—Novices tend to believe no one wants genetic counseling or supervision from the person wearing the "trainee badge" (Hendrickson et al., 2002).

Developmentally Based Interventions for Supervisors

Genetic counseling supervisors can use a variety of strategies to develop their knowledge and skills. As Callanan et al. (2016) note, these include

> trial and error, student feedback, consultation with colleagues, and drawing from one's own prior supervisors (Atzinger et al., 2014; Finley et al., 2016; Hendrickson et al., 2002; Lindh et al., 2003) . . . [and] training programs typically host annual (or more frequent) supervisor meetings that may involve . . . didactic content (e.g., supervision techniques and supervision dynamics). (p. 7)

Increasingly, supervision training is available at regional and national genetic counseling conferences as well.

One of the most powerful strategies is participation in ongoing peer supervision/consultation because it allows for focused time to reflect on one's supervision experiences, share perspectives, and give and receive support for this challenging activity (Lewis, Erby, et al., 2017; Zahm et al., 2016). Peer supervision (see Chapter 15) is an excellent resource for supervisors at all developmental levels and can be part of general mentorship in genetic counseling. In addition, some genetic counseling programs may require novice supervisors to have a supervision mentor. Boxes 5.2 and 5.3 contain additional cognitive and behavioral strategies for navigating novice and advanced stages of supervisor development, respectively.

BOX 5.2 Navigating Stages of Supervisor Development

Recommendations for Novice Supervisors

- Examine and draw from your own professional development and experiences as a supervisee.
- Think about the similarities and differences between your genetic counseling practice and your supervision practice, and extrapolate useful skills from your counseling work.
- Draw upon models of good supervision provided by supervisors in your own training.
- Engage in co-supervision with a colleague, if feasible.
- Participate in a peer supervision group.
- Pursue one-on-one mentorship with a more experienced supervisor.
- Establish and maintain clear boundaries with students.
- Address your novice status directly with students, and discuss any of their reactions.
- Remind yourself that you have more experience than students and more objectivity regarding their genetic counseling situations.
- Recognize that you may be especially able to establish a strong working alliance with students because you are close enough to your own graduate training to remember what it felt like to be a student.
- Don't be afraid to engage in trial and error as you develop and refine your style.
- Don't apologize for your novice status. You have a great deal to offer. And research supports the value of being a novice. For instance, studies of behavioral modeling suggest the most effective models are those who appear to be slightly ahead in their performance compared to "experts" whose skills may be perceived as unattainable by novice learners.

Adapted from Polanski, P. (2000, Winter). Training supervisors at the master's level: Developmental considerations. *ACES Spectrum Newsletter*, 3–5.

BOX 5.3 Navigating Stages of Supervisor Development

Recommendations for Advanced Supervisors

Acknowledge and Appreciate Your Strengths

- Having supervised multiple students, you have a foundation for knowing what to expect and recognizing when something seems "out of the norm" for a student and your supervision relationship.
- You can more quickly and easily discern the essential issues and needs of clients and supervisees.
- You have accrued a great deal of "muscle memory," and therefore you usually are more focused and efficient in your supervision work.

Work on Managing Common Challenges

- Your ability to quickly discern essential issues and needs may seem to some students (especially novices) that you make snap judgments and/or arrive at premature conclusions. It is important to explain to students the steps you only appear to bypass in coming to your conclusions. This can be difficult to do if you are not used to describing your process at such a granular level.
- Some students may feel intimidated because of your deep experience, knowledge, and skills. They may feel as if they could never reach your level of expertise. Conversely, some students may see how seamlessly you function as a genetic counselor and supervisor and think the work is easy.
- Beware of letting your preferred supervisory style become quicksand. Self-reflection, consultation, and openness to learning new things and trying different approaches can help keep you (and your students) on solid ground. Stagnation is one of the quickest ways to lose the gratification and effectiveness that come from working in an engaged, authentic, and responsive way.

Developmentally Based Interventions for Students

Several behavioral strategies may assist you in helping students develop professionally.

Engage in Assessment

An initial step in promoting student growth is to assess their general level of development. You could review with a student the evaluation forms you will use for the rotation and ask the student to evaluate themself on each item (e.g., I have not been trained in using this skill; I seldom use this skill; I use this skill often; I am comfortable using this skill; I am uncomfortable using this skill; I would like more information and training on this skill [Fall & Sutton, 2004, p. 13]). Pay attention to how a student approaches this activity: Are they confident? Uncertain? Are they able to provide examples of having achieved a particular skill? Do they express confusion about the meaning of a particular skill? Over time, observe their behavior to determine the accuracy of their self-appraisal.

Role plays comprise another way to assess a student's developmental level, allowing you to determine the extent to which they are able to apply their academic knowledge in actual practice. Role plays also help determine the accuracy of a student's evaluation of their skills.

Think about strategies you use to assess client understanding of information. How might you adapt those strategies to assess student developmental level?

Match Interventions to Developmental Level

Supervisors should select approaches to support a student's current developmental level while also providing sufficient challenge to encourage further development (Behavioral Health

Providers Association of New Mexico, 2021). Novice students tend to be dependent on and prefer high support and high direction from supervisors, whereas advanced students tend to prefer lower support and direction because they are more self-reliant. For example, using Stoltenberg and McNeill's (2011) IDM, supervisors working with a Level 1 student would be "supportive and prescriptive" in order to respond to high anxiety and dependence; for Level 3, they would "emphasize supervisee autonomy and engage in collegial challenging" (Behavioral Health Providers Association of New Mexico, 2021).

Use Examples

Regardless of developmental level, one of the most powerful tools for promoting learning and subsequent development consists of presenting concepts and skills in multiple ways and/or having students engage with concepts and skills in multiple tasks (D. Langley, personal communication, January 8, 2010). Examples concretize and deepen learning and can include analogies, demonstrations, diagrams/drawings, trial and error, photographs, problems, stories/narratives/scenarios, verbal descriptions, and videos (D. Langley, personal communication, January 8, 2010).

Assign Scaffolding Tasks/Experiences

Venne and Coleman (2010) suggest ways to structure learning that promotes development for genetic counseling students who are primarily either "risk adverse" (afraid to take chances, self-protective) or highly confident (seeking challenges that may eclipse their skill level). Although these authors write specifically about millennial students, I regard their ideas as relevant for all student supervisees. They recommend an "experiential evolutionary scaffolding" approach in which supervisors add increasingly complex tasks/experiences as students develop. There are three progressive stages of evolutionary scaffolding—expert, reciprocal, and self-scaffolding—in which control of a task shifts from external sources to internal, student-centered processes:

> *Expert scaffolding* (external supervisor-directed): Prevalent in fieldwork rotations, expert scaffolding involves the supervisor assessing a student's knowledge and the extent to which the student can apply this knowledge in real-world situations. Based on this assessment, the supervisor assigns specific activities to bridge the gap between knowledge and application (e.g., observation of role models, questions to promote student's critical thinking, and suggested readings). Imitation of the supervisor is a prevalent activity.
>
> *Reciprocal scaffolding* (mutually directed): The student and supervisor collaborate on tasks, often switching back and forth in the expert and learner roles. Reciprocal scaffolding is likely to occur, for instance, when a student finds empirical evidence during case prepping that the supervisor does not yet know.
>
> *Self-scaffolding* (internal student-directed): As students build their skills, they are better able to accurately self-evaluate, think critically about client needs, and independently determine how to address those needs (e.g., how to tailor a case prep for a given client). "Under self- scaffolding, the supervisor takes the position that the student learns more by doing even though it may make the student feel uncomfortable and less safe" (Venne & Coleman, 2010, p. 559).

An important aspect of the scaffolding process is provision of "support tools" until students can demonstrate and use a skill independently. Support tools in genetic counseling may include, among others, directing students to written resources, giving students examples of case preps and follow-up letters, co-counseling with clear delineation of the students' responsibilities during the session, and prepping and debriefing cases with students. The three types of scaffolding are briefly described next.

Venne and Coleman (2010) note that when genetic counseling supervisors begin with expert scaffolds, move to reciprocal ones, and finish with self-scaffolds, they "will provide shelter in earlier periods and build confidence that leads to achievement throughout the process" (p. 560). I suggest you explain scaffolding stages to students to help address common questions such as "What am I expected to be able to do now? By the end of the rotation?" Your explanation may also help offset the impatience some students feel when you initially assign expert scaffolding tasks: "The confident [students] do not want to constantly create outlines or conduct other mimicry tasks that seem designed to simply show that they know how to do something when they've once demonstrated that ability" (p. 562).

Examples of experiences you can modify to provide any of the three scaffolding stages include providing students with opportunities to observe sessions throughout the rotation; recording yourself (with a client or role playing with a colleague) and instructing students to watch and analyze the session independently or together; independently preparing a case prep and/or follow-up and then having the student compare/contrast their case prep/letter to yours; conducting mini role plays to show students what you expect and/or help them get a sense of how to implement a skill(s) with which they are struggling; video recording students' counseling interactions (real or role plays) so they (and you) can review and critique their skills; allowing students to do portions of a session from the "get go," and increasing the portions as their skills develop; giving students assignments that require self-appraisal between sessions.

Novices may participate in scaffolding tasks at a highly imitative level, whereas more advanced students will be better able to critically reflect upon the tasks and be more individualistic in how they approach them. Student variations in this regard are analogous to cooking, where novices follow a recipe to the letter, whereas advanced students use it as a general guide as they improvise ingredients and/or cooking procedures.

The next section discusses an experience that is the "ultimate" in self-scaffolding—counseling independently.

Counseling Independently

Promotion of student independent practice is one of the major outcomes of the Reciprocal-Engagement Model of Supervision (Wherley et al., 2015; see Chapter 1, this volume). For most students, it is important to have some experience with independent practice while still receiving supervision before graduating and practicing entirely on their own. The activities discussed next will promote student success in this undertaking.

Assess Student Readiness

Assessment of student readiness is an initial step toward independent practice. What do/would you look for to determine a student is ready to counsel independently? Box 5.4 lists various counseling behaviors and personal qualities that research (Hill et al., 2017, pp. 18, 26) suggests are indicative of readiness.

Several strategies can help you assess student readiness:

- Create a checklist of the behaviors and qualities listed in Box 5.4 and use it to assess your students on a weekly basis.
- Role play a portion of a session as part of case prep to determine what the student might be able to handle on their own.
- Instruct the student to role play a session with a classmate or with you and record the session. Review the role play to determine their skill level.
- Record an actual or simulated session and have the student critique their performance—either with you or independently (the student could transcribe the session and write a critique).

BOX 5.4 Factors Indicating Student Readiness to Counsel Independently

Counseling Behaviors

- Perceives comprehensive, meaningful patterns in information (e.g., client's psychosocial responses, family history information)
- Has adequate short- and long-term memory for relevant information during a session and in future sessions.
- Can execute basic skills/conduct the session in a timely manner
- Spends time developing ways to understand problems
- Represents client and counseling issues at a deep as opposed to a surface level
- Uses self-monitoring skills effectively
- Able to conceptualize clients
- Understands client dynamics
- Understands clinical ramifications of client situations
- Sees their interactions with clients in complex ways
- Understands the relationships among counseling techniques
- Develops management plans
- Values cognitive complexity and ambiguity
- Draws on accumulated experiences

Personal Qualities

- Grounded
- Comfortable in their own skin
- Self-aware
- Self-controlled
- Non-defensive
- Caring/compassionate
- Positive about self and others
- Easily develops warm and caring connection with clients while maintaining appropriate boundaries

- Dedicated to their own growth and to clients' welfare
- Sensitive
- Flexible
- Genuinely curious about clients

Source: Hill, C. E., Spiegel, S. B., Hoffman, M. A., Kivlighan, D. M., Jr., & Gelso, C. J. (2017). Therapist expertise in psychotherapy revisited. *The Counseling Psychologist, 45*, 7–53.

This strategy would allow you to assess their self-awareness and ability to self-evaluate accurately.

- During debriefings, assess the student's "mindfulness" by asking the student what they were aware of regarding their internal and external experiences as they occurred in the session. During actual sessions, watch for evidence that the student is giving their full attention to "being present" with clients (Hill et al., 2017, p. 27).
- Ask students their thoughts and feelings about counseling independently. If they express reluctance, ask them to specify their concerns to determine if you think the concerns are valid and, if so, ask them what they believe they need to do to address those concerns.

Prepare Students to Counsel Independently

The following strategies can help move students toward counseling independently:

- Begin the rotation with a clear expectation that students initially may "imitate" you but will work toward gradually incorporating more of their own style.

- Discuss how even when imitating, students will be developing their own style if they reflect upon how your approach fits/ does not fit for them.
- Encourage students to analyze/reflect on what you do and why you do it.
- As mentioned previously in this chapter, assign students small portions of the session where they can "do their own thing"; increase the portions as their skills progress.
- Write agendas with students for cases they conduct independently (i.e., a plan for how to conduct the session).
- Instruct students to include in a case prep the major goals for the session and five key points they wish to cover with the client. Have students use the key points as a mental or actual checklist during the session.
- Step in during the final minutes of a session to review with the client the key points and the extent to which these were covered.
- Discuss how students feel about attempting to counsel independently. What are they imagining to be the best outcome? The worst outcome?
- Reassure them the "worst outcome" seldom occurs and strategize what they could do if they should get stuck and/or feel overwhelmed (e.g., step out and find you).
- Some students may have perfectionistic expectations, and you will need to "push them" a bit to counsel independently.

Prepare Yourself for Students to Counsel Independently

One of the most important steps toward counseling independently begins with us as supervisors. When we use self-scaffolds, we give students more control over their practice. Relinquishing control requires us to tolerate the ambiguity of not knowing what students may say or do next. I recommend you examine your feelings and thoughts about independent student practice. If you feel reluctant about this experience, try to understand the cause(s) of your hesitancy: Is the student truly not ready? Do you doubt your assessment of their readiness? Are you afraid you would be unable to rectify any errors on their part? Is your investment in your clients making you overly cautious about allowing students to try counseling on their own? Are there other reasons? Discussion with peers may help you identify and manage these reasons.

Closing Thoughts

In closing, I pass along excellent advice from a social work supervisor (Moncho, 2013, para. 11) that is applicable for genetic counseling students and supervisors at all developmental levels. This advice highlights the importance of self-disclosure in supervision:

> Don't be afraid to say that you don't understand something, don't know how to do something, or wouldn't know what to do in a given situation. Keeping quiet because you're afraid of how you'll be perceived does no one any good, and what you don't know will eventually show up in your work anyway . . . get yourself out in front of the learning curve; make proactive learning a career-long habit. I have more confidence in and respect for a [person] who asks for the help they need, than for someone who plays it cool and drops the ball later—hopefully not to the detriment of [the client/supervisee].

Learning Activities

Most learning activities can be adapted for dyad or small group discussions or for written exercises. Time estimates are provided for discussions, but additional time should be allotted for large group processing.

Activity 5.1 Supervisor Development Self-Reflection

With a partner, discuss the following questions:

- What would someone say "stands out"/will stand out about how you practice as a supervisor? What is it that is particularly effective about how you supervise/will supervise?
- To what extent has that "distinguishing aspect" always been true of you versus something you have developed over time? What do you think contributed to your development of it?
- Some authors have described advanced supervisors as not only *master supervisors* but also *master genetic counselors*. What is your reaction to this perspective?

Estimated time: 15 minutes

Note: If you process this discussion in the larger group, I suggest focusing on the third question and asking whether any participants wish to share their responses to the first two questions.

Activity 5.2 Supervisor Development Self-Assessment

Prepare a written response to the following and then share your responses with a partner or in small groups:

- Using one of the stage models presented in this chapter, indicate which stage/phase best characterizes where you generally are in your development of supervisor competencies.
- Do you possess specific characteristics/skills that you would associate with a different stage(s) of development? [*Hint*: You may wish to refer to Eubanks Higgins et al. (2013) supervisor

competencies presented in Chapter 1, Appendix 1A for ideas about characteristics and skills.]

- *Supervisors only*: Think about a recent supervisee and, using the IDM of student development, describe the student's characteristics/skills suggestive of the stages of that model. [*Hint*: Most students will evidence behaviors indicative of more than one stage.]
- Do you generally prefer/think you would prefer to supervise novice, intermediate, or advanced students? Please explain.

Estimated time: 40 minutes

Activity 5.3 Experiential Evolutionary Scaffolding

With a partner or in small groups, identify a task you could assign a student for each stage of scaffolding (expert, reciprocal, and self-scaffolding) for each of the following activities [*Hint*: In determining the tasks, consider nuances such as taking less time, tailoring an approach to clients with different characteristics, anticipating client issues, etc.]:

- Prepare for a case
- Take a family history
- Explain the results of a genetic test to a client
- Describe an amniocentesis procedure
- Explain a variant of uncertain significance
- Document session in chart and/or in letter to a client

Estimated time: 45 minutes

Activity 5.4 Addressing Student Developmental Issues: Triad Role Plays

Take turns as supervisor, student, and observer for the following scenarios. After each role play, the student and observer should indicate what developmental issue(s) they thought the supervisor recognized and how they addressed the issues with the student.

Scenario 1

A novice student is very eager to impress you. They are so eager to show you how smart and thorough they think they are that they come to you about everything. They have been stopping by your office and sending you multiple emails. How would you address this with them?

Adapted from Moncho, C. (2013, August 10). *Structuring supervision*. The Social Work Practitioner. Retrieved January 21, 2021, from https://thesocialworkpractitioner.com/2013/08/10/structuring-supervision

Scenario 2

You and your intermediate student just finished a counseling session in which the client seemed ambivalent about genetic testing. Your student missed this and instead seemed to be pushing the client to go through with testing. You intervened and were able to explore the client's ambivalence. You are now debriefing the session and bring up how the student missed the client's ambivalence and what you said and did to address it with the client. Your student becomes increasingly withdrawn and quiet. When you ask them about this, they say they are pretty discouraged about their counseling skills and feel like giving up.

Scenario 3

Your intermediate student has begun their first rotation in cancer counseling. You assigned them a case prep for a client with a family history that includes multiple relatives with colon cancer and other cancers suggestive of Lynch syndrome or other colorectal cancer syndrome. You reviewed the case prep and see the student failed to make connections between the cancer diagnoses in the family and potential hereditary syndromes. When you point this out, they say, "but I worked really hard on this prep."

Scenario 4

You and your novice student just finished a prenatal counseling session in which the student took the family history. During the history taking, the client disclosed that she had several miscarriages but did not elaborate. Your student stopped looking at their checklist, made a statement about how difficult that must have been for the client, and then sat silently until she spoke again. You think your student handled this very well, but during debriefing they apologize, saying they are sorry for "going off script" and using up valuable session time.

Estimated time: 45 minutes

Note: This can be a written exercise in which participants construct a dialogue, formulating five student statements and five supervisor statements for each scenario.

Activity 5.5 Supervisor and Student Developmental Stages

With a partner or in small groups, discuss the following questions:

- What do you think are some of the potential benefits and challenges of having . . .
  - a novice student supervised by a novice supervisor?
  - an advanced student supervised by a novice supervisor?
  - a novice student supervised by an advanced supervisor?
  - an advanced student supervised by an advanced supervisor?
- How would you suggest a novice supervisor address with a novice student the fact that this is their first time supervising? With an advanced student?

Estimated time: 30 minutes

Note: The questions in the last bulleted point can also be role-played.

Setting Goals in Supervision

PATRICIA MCCARTHY VEACH

Objectives

- Describe the functions of goals in the supervision setting.
- Identify characteristics of viable goals.
- Suggest strategies for effectively setting goals.

A goal properly set is halfway reached.

—ZIG ZIGLAR (EVERYDAY POWER, N.D.)

What Are Goals and Why Are They Useful?

A *goal* is "the object of a person's ambition or effort; an aim or desired result," and it is synonymous with terms such as aim, objective, and purpose (English Oxford Living Dictionary, n.d.).[1] Goals serve several functions in supervision. They clarify what a supervisor expects of a student and provide a framework for the supervision relationship, the student's learning activities, and learning

---

1. Portions of this chapter are from McCarthy Veach (2021). Goal setting in genetic counseling supervision: Basic concepts and skills module. In *Supervision of genetic counseling students: How and why*. Association of Genetic Counseling Program Directors. http://media.mycrowdwisdom.com.s3.amazonaws.com/nsgc/Supervision%20Modules/scormcontent/index.html

outcomes (McCarthy Veach & LeRoy, 2009). Setting goals "causes one to think seriously and deeply about what is worth teaching" and requires a supervisor to answer the question: "What would anyone have to know or be able to do before being ready to practice this entire [genetic counseling] task?" (Mager, 1997, pp. 19, 39).

Goals help focus the work of supervision and student learning efforts by defining the number and type of skills that will take center stage (R. Curtis, 2000). Goals decrease student anxiety because they establish learning milestones, place limits on what seems like a limitless environment, prevent student–supervisor conflict by providing a road map of the learning process and expected destination, provide a yardstick against which to evaluate student performance, facilitate student self-evaluation (Fall & Sutton, 2004), and help students "balance self-improvement goals with client outcome goals" (R. Curtis, 2000, p. 204). Goal setting also models ways for students to effectively engage in this activity with their clients (R. Curtis, 2000; Wherley et al., 2015).

Types of Performance Goals

Goals vary with respect to how observable they are (Mager, 1997). *Visible* goals contain overt behaviors. They include, for example, creating a case preparation outline, drawing a pedigree, giving information to clients, and writing a follow-up letter. *Invisible* goals refer to covert or internal processes involving cognition and affect. Examples include knowing a risk rate, recognizing client feelings, understanding how a client might react when they receive a positive test result, and being aware of one's own thoughts and feelings when clients cry. Assessing progress on invisible goals is challenging unless you can connect the goals to visible behaviors you expect a student to demonstrate. Mager (1997) notes that indicators of an invisible goal "should be simple and direct" (p. 77). For example:

- An indicator for knowing a risk rate might be "State an accurate risk rate for *X* condition."
- An indicator for recognizing client feelings might be "State two feelings the client was experiencing during the session."

BOX 6.1 Ten Criteria for Viable Goals

Viable goals are . . .

- Set early in the supervision relationship
- Explicit rather than implicit
- Specific and clearly worded
- Feasible regarding capacity, opportunity, and resources
- Require supervisees to *stretch* themselves
- Related to the task formulated
- Modifiable over time
- Measurable
- Ordered by priority
- Mutually agreed upon (when possible)

Characteristics of Viable Goals

Viable goals contain three components: (1) the performance desired ("What do I want the student to be able to know, understand, do?"); (2) the conditions under which the performance should occur ("What are the important conditions or constraints under which I want them to perform?"); and (3) the level of skill required ("How well must the student perform for me to be satisfied?") (Mager, 1997). Box 6.1 contains a list of criteria for viable goals.

SMART is a widely known acronym representing several goal criteria. The SMART acronym stands for specific, measurable, attainable, relevant, and time-bound (agreed-upon time frame for goal accomplishment) (MacLeod, 2012).

Goal-Setting Processes

Goal setting is a process, not an event, and it is an essential part of supervision (Eubanks Higgins et al., 2013). In a study of genetic counselor supervisors (Suguitan et al., 2019), participants said goal-setting processes start at the beginning of the supervision relationship with contracting for the general goals of the rotation. They also described goal setting as occurring daily in planning discussions about each case (e.g., Participant: "This is probably what you're going to have to do. This is what you need to get ready in order to see that patient or to see a new diagnosis. Do everything you need to do and everything you need to know about that condition . . . [I] spell it out for each student" [Suguitan et al., 2019, p. 608]). Goal setting continues during case debriefings (e.g., Participant: "If they keep asking me, 'What should I do as follow up?' Without any grace I say, 'What do you think you should do as follow-up? . . . What do you feel like you still need to work on? Alright, let's have that be your follow-up to this case" [Suguitan et al., 2019, p. 608]).

Determining Goal Content

Determination of goal content addresses two of Mager's (1997) components of viable goals—the performance desired and conditions under which the performance will occur. There are many potential sources for deciding which skills and associated behaviors to prioritize and make the focus of supervision. Sources include, among others, the Accreditation Council for Genetic Counseling's (2019a) practice-based competencies; genetic counseling program expectations (often apparent in programs' evaluation forms); expectations of the rotation site; models of genetic counseling practice, such as the Reciprocal-Engagement Model (REM) (McCarthy Veach et al., 2007); generic counseling skills models, such as the Discrimination Model (Bernard, 1979, 1997; Lanning, 1986); and feedback/evaluations from prior rotations (based on student self-report and/or a collated statement from the student's program). Usually, you will draw upon more than one source when setting goals with students.

The Discrimination Model

The Discrimination Model offers a simple and comprehensive classification system for skills and behaviors pertinent to all types of genetic counseling goals. Bernard (1979, 1997) created this widely cited model to classify counseling skills into three broad categories: intervention, conceptualization, and personalization, and Lanning (1986) expanded the model by adding a professional skills category. The categories are defined as follows:

> *Intervention skills* are "doing skills." They include overt (observable) behaviors (strategies, techniques, and actions) students engage in when providing genetic counseling services.
>
> *Conceptualization* skills are "thinking skills." They include covert (invisible) behaviors related to internal processes of deliberate, strategic thinking and analysis about genetic counseling cases. Conceptualization skills allow students to connect their interventions to underlying principles (Australian Institute of Professional Counsellors [AIPC], 2019).
>
> *Personalization skills* are "feeling skills" that include the interface between a student's personal characteristics and their genetic counseling work, ability to form a counselor identity/style, and their subjective reactions during genetic counseling sessions and supervision interactions (AIPC, 2019). They also include self-regulatory skills, self-reflection skills, and the ability to learn from experience (AIPC, 2019). Behaviors related to personalization skills can be both overt and covert.
>
> *Professional skills* are overt "doing skills" pertaining to adherence to professional and ethical standards and behaviors. They also include behaviors generally accepted as professional (e.g., following the clinic dress code) (AIPC, 2019).

Box 6.2 contains examples of the four skills categories as applied to genetic counseling.

Establishing Goal Levels: Bloom's Taxonomy

Establishment of goal levels addresses Mager's (1997) third component of viable goals—the level of skill required. Genetic counseling

BOX 6.2 Examples of Skills Based on the Discrimination Model

Intervention Skills

- Explain the purpose of the genetic counseling session clearly, accurately, and succinctly.
- Have nonverbal facial expressions that are appropriate to the situation.
- Use open-ended questions to draw out client thoughts and feelings.
- Use silence appropriately.
- Appropriately use information that comes out in the session.
- Present information in an organized manner.

Conceptualization Skills

- Understand how people with the same conditions may need to be worked with differently.
- Conceptualize client needs accurately.
- Prioritize client needs appropriately.
- Identify plans that are specific and appropriate for clients.
- Choose and apply responses in sessions that are appropriate and timely.
- Interpret client behaviors accurately.

Personalization Skills

- Are aware of personal needs for approval from the client and/or supervisor.
- Maintain a nonjudgmental attitude despite value differences.
- Identify and manage personal feelings generated in clinical interactions.
- Effectively manage own frustrations about lack of progress in skill development.
- Are aware of their level of comfort with uncertainty.
- Receive feedback non-defensively.

Professional Skills

- Maintain appropriate relationships with peers, supervisors, and other colleagues.
- Maintain client confidentiality.
- Take advantage of additional opportunities for training.
- Seek consultative help as needed.
- Adhere to clinic charting policies.

Adapted from Lanning, W. (1986). Development of the supervisor emphasis rating form. *Counselor Education & Supervision, 25,* 191–196.

goals should specify the desired degree of cognitive and behavioral complexity expected of students. Bloom's Taxonomy of educational objectives (Bloom et al., 1956) is a classic framework for establishing goal levels. Bloom describes six levels of increasing complexity. Table 6.1 contains a description of the levels and an example of each.

Goal-Setting Strategies

Goal setting is an ongoing, interactive process involving different "working parts." This section contains several strategies for enhancing that process.

Establish Long- and Short-Term Goals

Long-term goals are the outcomes desired by the end of the rotation, and they tend to be fairly broad (R. Curtis, 2000). In addition to overall objectives established by the rotation site, long-term goals should relate to a student's current developmental level and

TABLE 6.1 Bloom's Taxonomy of Levels and Examples

Level	Description and Example
Knowledge	Recall or recognize appropriate facts, concepts, principles. List, repeat, memorize, recall, state. *List the steps involved in an amniocentesis procedure.*
Comprehension	Translate, interpret, extrapolate. *Interpret a pedigree to identify an individual who is at high risk for cardiomyopathy.*
Application	Use facts, concepts, and principles in a hypothetical or real situation. Illustrate, demonstrate, employ, give an example. *Describe the steps in an ultrasound procedure in a way that the patient can understand.*
Analysis	Compare/contrast, deduce, dissect, break down. *Compare and contrast the likely response to prophylactic procedures for a 25-year-old versus a 50-year-old woman at risk for breast cancer.*
Synthesis	Integrate, consolidate, build, join. *Consolidate data from client chart, parent self-report, and relevant literature on fragile X to discuss possible long-term consequences for their child.*
Evaluation	Critique, assess, judge, debate, determine the worth of. *Assess client likely reaction to positive genetic test result and modify session as needed.*

Adapted from Bloom, B. S., Englehart, M. D., Furst, E. J., Hill, W. H., & Krathwohl, D. R. (1956). *Taxonomy of educational objectives: Handbook I. cognitive domain.* McKay.

needs (see Chapter 5). Examples include gaining a stronger professional identity, growing in confidence, functioning more autonomously, and self-evaluating accurately. You should identify long-term goals at the beginning of the supervision relationship.

Short-term goals concern daily and weekly rotation experiences, include both students' and clients' needs (R. Curtis, 2000), and tend to be more specific. Short-term goals emerge primarily from case preparations and session debriefings, and they help ensure you and the student are on the "same page." Examples include managing pediatric sessions when children are present; becoming comfortable working with an interpreter in sessions; and explaining positive, negative, or ambiguous test results.

Regularly Review Long- and Short-Term Goals

Discussing goals as the rotation progresses will yield more focused and precise learning priorities. I suggest you review long-term goals at least weekly to assess student progress and decide whether any goals require modification. Review of short-term goals typically occurs more often, during case planning and session debriefing. As part of case planning, decide on one or two goals to pay particular attention to during each counseling session. Then during debriefings, discuss the student's perspective and your impressions of the extent to which they achieved each goal. This discussion may lead to modified and/or new goals for future sessions.

Make Goal Setting a Collaborative and Focused Process

I feel like students are often either unclear on their learning priorities, or have trouble verbalizing them.

GENETIC COUNSELOR SUPERVISOR
(AS CITED IN FINLEY ET AL., 2016, P. 350)

Create a Working Draft

Ask students to write down their goals and bring them to your first meeting. Set a limit on the number of those goals—two or three. R. Curtis (2000) notes that although "beginning counselors may not know all of the appropriate areas in which to set goals . . . having them think about their goals early in the [rotation] makes them aware that the supervision process will be purposeful" (p. 202). This strategy can also provide you with insight into the student's self-assessment of their skills and learning priorities.

Use a Goal-Setting Rubric

Consider using a simple form (see Learning Activity 6.2) to work with students on turning learning priorities into behavioral goal statements.

Ask the Miracle Question

The miracle question is a psychotherapy technique for encouraging clients to focus on desirable behavior changes rather than on limitations and deficiencies. Adapted for supervision, the miracle question helps beginning counselors focus on positive outcomes (R. Curtis, 2000). Ask your students to imagine what they would like to be doing differently once they have completed the rotation. The miracle question encourages them to imagine themselves as capable genetic counselors and allows them to consider the skills necessary to do so (R. Curtis, 2000). If a student responds with a goal that seems more negative than positive, prompt them further. For instance,

> *Supervisor*: What would you like to be doing differently by the end of this rotation?
>
> *Student*: I'd like to be less nervous when I'm counseling clients.
>
> *Supervisor*: And what would "less nervous" look like?

Note that if you use this technique, do not refer to it as the "miracle question" because some students may think you are implying it would take a miracle for them to become skilled genetic counselors!

Modify Goals as Appropriate

It is not always clear what the learning needs are of the student until further along in the rotation when I have had experience seeing the issues that need to be worked on for that site.

—GENETIC COUNSELOR SUPERVISOR

(AS CITED IN FINLEY ET AL., 2016, P. 350)

Goals are dynamic; therefore, ongoing review and modification are an inherent part of the process. If you are able to gather information about a student's strengths and growth areas from their programs and/or self-report prior to beginning supervision, you may be able to more quickly pinpoint some of their learning needs. You might ask programs to encourage site supervisors to help students develop one or more specific goals for their next rotation.

Goals should "expand" as students develop their skills. Although the topic of a goal may remain the same, the expectation of performance should increase. For example, an initial goal may be for the student to take an accurate family history. Once the student demonstrates that ability with some consistency, the goal could expand to taking an accurate family history more efficiently (in less time). Once that goal is achieved, it might expand to collecting the history in a more interactive way (e.g., asking open-ended questions that elicit several details from clients).

Recognize and Manage Common Goal-Setting Pitfalls

Goals Based on Supervisor and/or Student Implicit Expectations

It is important to recognize and manage implicit expectations because they can damage the working alliance and hinder student learning and development. Honestly reflect on any unrealistic expectations you have about student performance (e.g., setting too many goals and/or not prioritizing them) and perfectionistic expectations (e.g., expecting a novice student to perform as well as the advanced student you recently supervised). Consciously put aside those expectations. Watch for indications of students' unspoken expectations (e.g., a novice student thinks they should be able to counsel an entire session alone by the third week of a rotation or an advanced student thinks it is okay to do "just enough to get by" because they dislike the specialty). Discuss their implicit expectations and how and why goals related to these expectations are not feasible.

Goals That Are Overly Focused on Ego or Task Orientations

R. Curtis (2000) describes two goal orientations—ego and task—and notes that people vary in their preferences for each orientation. Individuals who operate from a high ego–low task orientation tend to set implicit and explicit goals related to success or failure (based primarily on clients' reactions and behaviors). Students with this orientation are likely to be more anxious and have less self-confidence because they assess their ability solely on outcomes that are not always within their control. People with a high task–low ego orientation tend to emphasize and set goals related to self-improvement (based on self-assessment and others' assessment of their skill development). Their goals often are more realistic, and they "tend to use failure as a signal to reconsider their strategies or increase their effort" (p. 196).

Goal orientations have important implications for student development and the outcomes of the services they provide. Neither orientation should be minimized or be the exclusive focus when setting goals and evaluating goal attainment. I suggest you reflect on your own goal orientation and assess students' goal orientations to set goals that balance ego and task. As R. Curtis (2000) notes, "It is important for supervisors to help beginning counselors recognize their goal-setting tendencies so they can avoid unnecessary 'self-blame' pitfalls and concentrate on improving their skills" (p. 198). Finally, I recommend attending to the ways you discuss goal attainment throughout supervision, helping students discern the extent to which genetic counseling outcomes are due to their skill level versus factors outside their control. For example,

> Student: My goal for this rotation is to make sure clients leave feeling empowered. [ego-oriented goal]
>
> Supervisor: How a client feels when they leave may not be something you can control. What are some specific behaviors you can engage in to encourage a client to be empowered? [task-oriented goal]

Evaluate Your Goal-Setting Skills

Self-Evaluation

Finley et al. (2016) investigated genetic counseling supervisors' self-efficacy for 12 goal-setting competencies established by Eubanks Higgins et al. (2013) (e.g., *I can incorporate the student's developmental level into the rotation goals* and *I can set realistic learning goals through discussion with a student*). You can use the items and rating scale described in their article to evaluate your goal-setting self-efficacy. If your efficacy is lower for certain items, use those as growth points.

Student Evaluation

Invite student feedback about your goal-setting skills. Lehrman-Waterman and Ladany (2001) developed a scale for supervisees to evaluate supervisor goal-setting and feedback skills. Thirteen items assess goal setting (e.g., *My supervisor and I created goals which were easy for me to understand* and *I felt uncertain as to what my most important goals were for this training experience*). You could use some of these items to focus a conversation about the goal-setting process at the rotation mid-point (or earlier). You might also ask if students' programs could include this scale (with slight modification to some items to make them relevant to genetic counseling) when they collect end-of-rotation student feedback. Programs could send you collated results from a few supervisees across a period of time.

Strategies for Promoting Goal Accomplishment

Most goals provide an indication of desired *outcomes* regarding student development and performance. But goals in and of themselves do not always provide a clear bridge to the actions necessary to achieve those outcomes. Supervisors should help students identify specific *strategies* and *behaviors* to achieve these outcomes and inform them about how their efforts to achieve the goals will be *measured*. Box 6.3 contains examples of goals from the REM of genetic counseling practice (McCarthy Veach et al., 2007), select strategies and behaviors (Redlinger-Grosse et al., 2017), and measurement methods.

Mind Mapping

For a student who is having a lot of trouble, I find it difficult to have a conversation about changing her goals to something that may be easier to meet. I want to avoid crushing her spirits and making her feel that I don't think she can accomplish what we had originally discussed, since I feel this might make her do worse if she thinks I don't have faith in her.

—GENETIC COUNSELOR SUPERVISOR
(AS CITED IN FINLEY ET AL., 2016, P. 350)

Mind mapping is a creative brainstorming and planning technique to assist students in identifying ways to master strategies and

BOX 6.3 Examples of Goals, Strategies, Behaviors, and Measurement Methods

Goal: Creates a working contract with client
Strategy: Establish a working alliance
Behaviors: Asks open- and close-ended questions; reflects client experiences and feelings using primary empathy; uses attending skills (silence, eye contact, head nods)
Measured by: Live observation

Goal: Recognizes client strengths
Strategy: Assess client strengths
Behaviors: Asks close-ended questions about client's support system; asks open-ended questions about client's coping strategies; uses primary empathy to clarify/summarize client's strengths
Measured by: Live observation

Goal: Help client feel informed about the purpose of genetic counseling
Strategy: Gather information regarding client expectations of genetic counseling
Behaviors: Asks open-ended questions; summarizes client responses; provides corrective information regarding inaccurate expectations
Measured by: Case prep; live observation

Goal: Presents information in a way that clients can understand
Strategy: Assess client understanding of information
Behaviors: Draws out inheritance pattern for client; shows pictures; paces information presented based on client's non-verbal reactions
Measured by: Case prep; live observation

behaviors related to their goals. A mind map visually organizes steps (actions, resources, and experiences) that contribute to development of the desired strategy or behavior. Focusing on "smaller steps" often means the original goal(s) does not have to change.

The supervisor and student begin by listing the strategy in the center of the paper and then they draw lines (like the spokes of a wheel) around the strategy. Next, they collaboratively identify steps to achieve the strategy and list one step on each spoke. Figure 6.1 contains an example of a mind map for the strategy of managing couple conflict during a session.

Mind mapping has added benefits of helping students feel less overwhelmed by the perceived difficulty of a strategy and building self-confidence as they achieve individual steps. When using a mind mapping technique, I suggest you (1) ask the student to personally commit to taking the actions identified for achieving the strategy, (2) establish a timeline for accomplishing each action because this will promote ongoing progress, (3) watch for and discuss the student's success toward mastery of the strategy, and (4) revise or add action steps as appropriate.

Goal: Facilitate decision-making

Strategy: Manage prenatal couple conflict regarding decisions

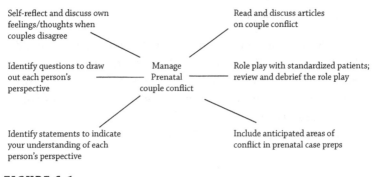

FIGURE 6.1

Mind mapping example.

Closing Thoughts

I encourage you to be systematic and selective in setting goals with students. It is not possible (and would be overwhelming) to give equal attention to every practice-based competency during a rotation. It is important to be realistic. "Some goals will need to be pursued before others, different goals will be of varying lengths, and some will not even come into view until [students have] moved on in [their] development" (AIPC, 2019). Goals are a road map to a final destination. They provide direction but require modification as you come upon roadblocks, shortcuts, and other sorts of "travel" conditions. Updating and referring regularly to your road map will help you and your student enjoy the trip to the desired destination.

Learning Activities

Most learning activities can be adapted for dyad or small group discussions or for written exercises. Time estimates are provided for discussions, but additional time should be allotted for large group processing.

Activity 6.1 Writing Viable Goals

In small specialty groups (prenatal, pediatric, cancer, lab, etc.), do the following:

- Write five goals reflecting skills you would want students to be able to demonstrate by a rotation's end in that specialty.
- Draw a circle around the performance in each goal statement to be sure you have stated a specific behavior/skill.
- Exchange your list of goals with another group and ask them what they think each one of your goals means.

[Hint: You may want to decide whether you are writing goals for a first rotation, mid-rotation, or final rotation student.]

Estimated time: 30 minutes

Note: Participants could share goals with several students and ask the students what they think each goal means.

Adapted from Mager, R. F. (1997). *Preparing instructional objectives* (3rd ed.). CEP Press.

Activity 6.2 Connecting Goals to Behaviors and Goal Measurement

In small groups, do the following:

Select a specific genetic counseling specialty and identify *three essential skills* (goals) for a novice student's (i.e., first rotation) performance.
   a. Using the Goal-Setting Grid below, list each skill.
   b. Identify up to *three target behaviors* that would demonstrate accomplishment of each skill.
   c. Describe how a supervisor would measure student performance of each behavior.
   d. Repeat steps b and c for each intermediate students and for advanced students.

[*Hint*: Some target behaviors and/or ways of measuring them may be the same, or they may differ across student experience levels.]

Goal-Setting Grid

   Example
      Skill: "Able to establish with clients a common agenda for the session."
      Target behavior (beginning student): Asks client why they are seeking genetic counseling.
      Measured by: Supervisor notes taken during counseling session about the target behavior.

Target behavior (intermediate student): Suggests additional agenda items that might be relevant for the client.

Measured by: Supervisor notes taken during counseling session about the target behavior.

Target behavior (advanced student): Reflects client reluctance to be at the session and how this reluctance makes it difficult to identify an agenda for the session.

Measured by: Supervisor notes taken during counseling session about the target behavior.

Skill #1	*Beginning Student*	*Intermediate Student*	*Advanced Student*
Target Behavior 1: Measured by:			
Target Behavior 2: Measured by:			
Target Behavior 3: Measured by:			

Repeat this grid for Skills 2 and 3.

Estimated time: 45 minutes

Note: If time is limited, each group can be assigned one student developmental level (i.e., novice, intermediate, or advanced).

Activity 6.3 Writing Goals Using the Discrimination Model and Bloom's Taxonomy

In small groups, do the following:

- Identify and list one skill for each of the four skill categories in the Discrimination Model.
- Write a goal statement for each skill that reflects each Bloom level.

You can refer to examples of the Discrimination Model and Bloom's Taxonomy provided in the chapter, but you should not limit yourself to those examples.

Discrimination Model Skill Category	Bloom Level					
	Knowledge Goal	Comprehension Goal	Application Goal	Analysis Goal	Synthesis Goal	Evaluation Goal
Intervention skill (doing skill):						
Conceptualization skill (thinking skill):						
Personalization skill (feeling skill):						
Professional skill (adhering to professional standards skill):						

Estimated time: 45 minutes

Note: Groups can be assigned either based on specialty or randomly. If time is limited, each group can be assigned either one skill category or one Bloom level.

Activity 6.4 Mind Mapping to Promote Goal/Strategy Accomplishment

In small groups, do the following:

- Identify a genetic counseling goal and one strategy related to that goal.
- List the strategy in the center of the page.

- Draw spokes out from the center and fill each spoke with an action the student will take to work toward mastery of the strategy. Try to brainstorm a variety of steps (actions, resources, and experiences).
- Review each step to determine whether it should be broken into smaller steps.

[*Hint*: Refer to the example of a mind map in Figure 6.1 for help with creating your own.]

Estimated time: 20 minutes

Note: Groups can be assigned based either on specialty or randomly.

Activity 6.5 Setting and Prioritizing Short-Term Goals

Working individually, list three to five behaviors/actions that you regard as "must haves" with respect to student skill performance during typical sessions (e.g., *Student adequately addressed the client's questions*).
State the goal that corresponds to each behavior/action.
Then compare lists with a partner or in small groups.

Estimated time: 30 minutes

Note: This activity can promote supervisor reflection on the goals they consider to be priorities in genetic counseling sessions. They can communicate these priorities to students and use them to focus feedback during debriefings. This could also be used as a student activity.

7

Giving and Receiving Feedback

PATRICIA MCCARTHY VEACH

Objectives

- Describe the function of feedback in supervision.
- Identify primary types of feedback.
- Present strategies for promoting helpful feedback interactions.

Words are singularly the most powerful force available to humanity. We can choose to use this force constructively with words of encouragement, or destructively using words of despair. Words have energy and power with the ability to help, to heal, to hinder, to hurt, to harm, to humiliate and to humble.

—YEHUDA BERG (AS CITED IN COGNOLOGY, N.D.)

Feedback is one of the most frequent and consequential clinical supervision activities. Feedback is essential for achieving the purposes of genetic counseling supervision, namely promoting students' skill development and skill maintenance, ensuring a standard of care for clients, and helping determine whether students have gained the necessary skills to be a genetic counselor.

"The importance of feedback likely derives from its status as one of the few measures of progress available to students" (MacFarlane, 2013, p.189). Feedback is a *formative evaluation* method, providing ongoing review and discussion of students' skills, attitudes, behaviors, and appearance (Hoffman et al., 2005).

Genetic counseling supervisors and students highly value feedback, yet it is one of the most challenging supervision skills (Hendrickson et al., 2002; MacFarlane et al., 2016; McCarthy Veach et al., 2009). Fortunately, however, feedback skills can improve with deliberate practice.

Feedback is an important skill for evaluating student performance, the supervision relationship, and supervision processes (Martin et al., 2014). This chapter primarily addresses feedback about student performance, but the concepts and strategies presented herein are relevant for any aspect of supervision.

Types of Feedback

There are two primary types of feedback—positive feedback and corrective feedback.

Positive Feedback

Positive feedback involves identification and communication of behavior the supervisor wishes the student to continue and/or increase. For example, the supervisor says, "You waited for the client to speak after you told him the test result before you said anything further. I think that worked well. What are your thoughts about why it was effective?"

Reflection Questions for Readers: Have you ever refrained from giving someone positive feedback? If so, why was that?

Supervisors may fail to provide positive feedback to students for several reasons (McCarthy Veach et al., 2009):

- Forgetting that students need to hear encouraging comments to support their efforts, bolster their self-confidence, and direct their attention to their successes, however small they may be.
- Prioritizing corrective feedback over positive feedback, particularly if time is limited.
- Fearing their feedback will seem gratuitous. Supervisors and/or students may take certain skills for granted—for instance, thinking everyone has good eye contact.
- Thinking the student might discount the feedback. Anxious students, in particular, may gloss over positive comments to get corrective feedback "over with."
- Worrying the student may become too dependent on the supervisor's approval.
- Viewing the student's performance *globally* rather than as discrete behaviors. For example, observing a student taking a family history and only noting it was disorganized overlooks specific things the student said and did that were skillful.
- Reserving positive feedback for perfect performance, which, of course, never occurs for anyone.

Corrective Feedback

Corrective feedback consists of identification and communication of behavior the supervisor wishes the student to decrease and/or eliminate as well as discussion of what the student might do to resolve the behavior. For example, the supervisor says,

> The client is not a native English speaker and told you she would be okay with English if you took things slowly. You gave her several important pieces of information about trisomy 18 all at once. She seemed to understand but looked like she was struggling to do so. How might you have made things a little easier for her?

Reflection Question for Readers: Do you ever use the term negative feedback?

People often refer to corrective feedback as *negative feedback*. If you look up *negative* in a thesaurus, you will see synonyms such as *bad* and *harmful*. I contend that most supervisors and students who use the term *negative* to denote corrective feedback may inadvertently communicate it is something to avoid. A different term might have a more favorable connotation. Some people use the term *constructive feedback* instead. Although this term is better than negative feedback, "the possible implication [is] that positive feedback is not constructive [and] may lead some students (and supervisors) to devalue it or not focus on it sufficiently" (MacFarlane, 2013, p. 194). Therefore, I suggest using the term *corrective feedback*.

Giving corrective feedback is challenging (Lindh et al., 2003). Some supervisors are uncomfortable giving corrective feedback and may even withhold certain feedback for any of several reasons (McCarthy Veach et al., 2009). These reasons are listed in Box 7.1.

Conversely, some supervisors provide excessive amounts of corrective feedback, usually at the expense of positive feedback (Hendrickson et al., 2002). Corrective feedback tends to cause a drop in a student's confidence and increases their anxiety (MacFarlane et al., 2016). These reactions are an expected and temporary aspect of a student's developmental process when feedback is balanced (positive and corrective) (see Chapter 5), but excessive corrective feedback in the absence of supportive positive feedback can severely hinder student development and damage the supervisory working relationship (Ramos-Sánchez et al., 2002). Students may still learn and build their skills, but the extent of their growth will be diminished, and they may approach future supervision relationships with a self-protective shell that continues to restrict their development.

BOX 7.1 Reasons Supervisors Are Uncomfortable Giving Corrective Feedback

- No one else has observed or commented on the behavior in question.
- The supervisor second guesses the validity of their feedback.
- The supervisor is concerned it might mean they are a *bad* supervisor because the student is making mistakes.
- The supervisor is unsure of what the student must do to address the behavior.
- They think the feedback might damage the supervision relationship.
- They are concerned about the student's reaction to the feedback. For example, the student might obsess about it, be closed to/defensive about the feedback, shut down and lose all self-confidence, and/or get angry.
- The supervisor worries that the student is too fragile to handle the feedback.
- The student might react by disliking the supervisor and/or giving a negative evaluation.
- In extreme cases, supervisors fear litigation.

Source: McCarthy Veach, P., Willaert, R., & LeRoy, B. S. (2009). *Giving and receiving feedback in supervision: A DVD workbook*. University of Minnesota, Minneapolis, MN.

Characteristics of Helpful Feedback

The two words "information" and "communication" are often used interchangeably, but they signify quite different things. Information is giving out; communication is getting through.
—SYDNEY J. HARRIS (AS CITED IN COGNOLOGY, N.D.)

Reflection Questions for Readers: Think about some positive feedback you received that was particularly helpful. What was it about the feedback that made it so helpful? Now think about some corrective feedback you received that was helpful. What made that feedback helpful?

For each type of feedback, you probably identified something about its *content* and something about the *feedback approach*. Supervisor and student stylistic preferences (consulting, directive teaching, evocative teaching, counseling, and evaluation; see Chapter 2) affect *what* is attended to during supervision (feedback content) and *how* it is attended to (feedback approach). Feedback content also arises from long- and short-term goals established in the supervision relationship (see Chapter 6).

Eubanks Higgins et al. (2013; see also Chapter 1, Appendix 1A) identified several genetic counseling supervisor feedback competencies. Feedback includes verbal and nonverbal supportive statements delivered in a timely manner and in a private location. Feedback is clear, specific, honest, and objective; appropriate to a student's level of development; and concerns modifiable behaviors rather than traits that cannot be changed. Feedback is a two-way process that includes supervisors asking students their thoughts and feelings about their skills (self-feedback), assessing understanding of feedback given to them, attending to students' attempts to address feedback, and noting their progress in that regard. A criterion not mentioned in the supervisor competencies is providing balanced feedback—supportive and challenging comments (Borders, 2014).

Strategies for Promoting Helpful Feedback Interactions

There are several cognitive and behavioral strategies you can use to create helpful feedback interactions. These strategies pertain to setting the stage for feedback, engaging in ongoing feedback, and evaluating feedback processes.

Create a Framework for Feedback

Discuss Feedback Processes

When beginning a supervision relationship, inform the student about when and how feedback generally occurs, your approach to feedback, how the student can request feedback, and your expectations regarding their responsiveness to feedback. Of note, research shows genetic counseling students have difficulty integrating feedback from different supervisors (MacFarlane et al., 2016)—a difficulty that can be compounded when they have multiple supervisors during a rotation. When this is the case, inform the student which supervisor will take the lead on helping them integrate disparate feedback (Chapter 14 addresses additional challenges of having multiple supervisors).

Suggest Strategies for Receiving Feedback

Encourage the student to work on making themself open and responsive to feedback by using the following strategies (McCarthy Veach & LeRoy, 2009): letting you know when they do not understand some part of the feedback; requesting specific feedback about issues of concern to them; valuing positive feedback as information about skills they can use deliberately in the future; expecting corrective feedback as a natural part of development and using it as motivation to try things differently; checking out with others feedback that does not seem to quite "fit," and working to understand which parts may be valid; sharing how they are feeling and thinking about feedback; and, if feeling overwhelmed, asking to continue the conversation at a later time.

Prepare Students for Step-Ins

Step-ins refer to instances when a supervisor takes over a task or conversation with the client during a session. Step-ins are a significant aspect of the feedback process. Inform the student about when and why you generally do step-ins, and ask the student to anticipate how they will feel about them. Establish a process for handing the session back to the student after a step-in (e.g., saying to the client "[name of student] will now talk to you about . . ."). Also discuss how you would like the student to let you know during counseling sessions if they need you to step in. Step-ins are an emotional experience for students because they are probably

> thinking about [your] evaluation of their performance... (and even receiving indirect feedback when [you] "step in" to correct [their] behavior). . . . Some students may find it particularly daunting to contemplate supervisor feedback while interacting with clients and then "re-experience" that feedback during session debriefings. (MacFarlane, 2013, p. 192)

Schedule Time for Distal Feedback

Lindh et al. (2003) found most genetic counseling supervisors frequently or always provide feedback as soon as a counseling session ends. This approach has several benefits: "Feedback directly after a session often focuses on intuitive reactions, correction of technical skills (e.g., correction of terminology), and counseling *micro skills* (e.g., use of silence)" (p. 37). Research shows that students appreciate immediate feedback (MacFarlane et al., 2016). Immediate feedback is also more efficient in that it reduces the time needed to recollect details when a session is discussed later.

Immediate feedback also has potential drawbacks. The feedback will be limited if each session becomes a "one and done"—that is, you do not make connections regarding patterns of student performance across clients. Thus, your focus will tend to be on micro skills, which, although important, do not explicitly connect to students' longer term goals and overall progress. As Lindh et al. (2003) note, "Distal feedback (e.g., 3–4 days later) allows the supervisor and student to be more reflective about the . . . session and to focus on *macro skills* such as student comfort with affect and sensitivity to cultural issues" (p. 37). Another limitation of immediate feedback is that students' initial reactions tend to be affective (e.g., *I messed up that explanation of X . . .; I'm glad my supervisor didn't take as many notes this time*); they may need more time to cognitively process what did and did not work. Novice students, in particular, may need more time to reflect on what merits discussion. As a genetic counseling student stated, "It feels like you zoomed through this [counseling session]. You have no idea what was good, what happened" (Hendrickson et al., 2002, p. 35). Consequently, feedback immediately after a session may be very supervisor-dependent and could turn into a monologue as opposed to a mutual discussion.

I suggest you schedule time for distal feedback—that is, broader discussion at some later point to allow for a more interactive and "bigger picture" discussion about patterns in the student's performance. A good time to schedule distal feedback meetings is at the beginning of the rotation when you set the stage for supervision.

Use Evocative Feedback Strategies When Feasible

A question has the most power before we rush to answer it, when it is still making us think, still testing us.

—WINSPEAR (2009, P. 96)

Evocative feedback strategies can result in a highly effective feedback process. Evocative strategies involve drawing out the student's perspective before sharing your own perspective. As noted in Chapter 2, an evocative approach involves *leading by following*. Evocative strategies create a norm of balanced and shared feedback that provides both support and direction and builds student self-reflective skills along with the skills that are the subject of the feedback. Thus, evocative strategies encourage self-supervision, increase student confidence about having more "answers" than they may have thought, and promote independent practice.

Inform students that you tend to use evocative strategies, explain why, and give them an example:

> Usually when we begin to discuss your performance, I will ask you to identify one thing you did that you thought went well and why, and one thing you thought did not go as well and why. Next, I will share my impressions of one thing that went well and one thing that did not go as well. Then, we'll work together to figure out what you might do differently.

Being upfront about this approach and its purpose will help prevent students' viewing it as a "quiz" about their performance.
Take your time. I'd rather have a thoughtful answer than a fast one.
—PENNY (2013, P. 38)

When a student says, "I can't think of anything," or "I don't know" to your evocative questions, unless a response is needed immediately (e.g., for the next counseling appointment that day), ask them to take some time to think about it on their own and then tell you their ideas the next time you meet. They will come up with some ideas on their own and/or ask a peer for input. Either way, this will increase their learning and confidence that although they may not know all the answers, they have the ability to find them.

Shape Students' Self-Critique Skills

Ask your student to identify one or two skills they want to focus on so that you can watch for these skills in counseling sessions. During debriefings, ask them to self-critique these skills and then provide your critique. Require your student to be balanced in their comments, including both strengths and areas for improvement.

When students ask you for feedback, encourage them to be specific ("When I explained _____ to the client, she seemed confused. Did I go over it too quickly?" versus "Were my explanations ok?").

Provide Timely Feedback

Genetic counseling student: I felt like I didn't really hear a whole lot [of feedback] during the semester, and then at the end of the semester evaluation I didn't get very high marks, and I was a little bit blindsided because . . . nobody had been talking to me along the way about these things.

—MACFARLANE ET AL. (2016, P. 761)

Supervised rotations are a critical setting for students to try out skills, make mistakes, and identify and resolve them. Corrective feedback must include time and opportunities whenever possible for students to modify their behavior. Informing a student about problematic behavior when it is too late for them to do anything about it quite simply is unfair.

Be Honest and Direct

Psychotherapy supervisor: If I hem and haw and try to protect the supervisee from learning what I need to say, it doesn't go as well.

—MCCARTHY VEACH ET AL. (2012, P. 218)

Would you ever give a client falsely reassuring information or withhold critical information? The same is true for providing positive and corrective feedback to students. You can and should tell students your impressions of their performance.

Relatedly, it is important to be honest about whether feedback is based on "right and wrong" (e.g., "The risk rate you have in your case prep is inaccurate. It should be . . .") versus "two rights"—that is, stylistic differences (e.g., "You should use the word *fetus*, not *baby* when talking with pregnant parents"). Stylistic differences may be acceptable provided the client receives a standard of care (McCarthy Veach & LeRoy, 2009), as illustrated in the following quote (Goodyear et al., 2017):

> Emil Zatopek, a triple gold medalist at the 1952 Olympics . . . was not a graceful runner. With every step his body rolled and heaved, his head lurched back and forth, and his tongue lolled out. . . . He was well-aware of his less-than-perfect style, saying, "I shall learn to have a better style once they start judging races according to their beauty. So long as it's a question of speed, my attention will be directed to seeing how fast I can cover ground." (pp. 57–58)

If clients are receiving a standard of care, then critiques of the "beauty" of the student's performance may be less crucial. When you decide to provide corrective feedback about a stylistic difference, it can be helpful to name it as such and couch it as "another approach to add to your skill repertoire." It is also important to explain to students the reason(s) for your stylistic preferences—that is, the clinical ramifications (McCarthy Veach et al., 2012).

Provide Sufficient, Balanced Feedback

Some students will perceive everything a supervisor does and does not say as feedback. When supervisors say little or nothing, students may misinterpret the silence, thinking either their performance was so good that nothing else needs to be said or it was so poor that the supervisor does not know where to begin to discuss it. Furthermore, although corrective feedback, in particular, may be difficult to hear, students feel cheated and struggle when supervisors fail to engage fully in feedback. As one genetic counseling student said (as cited in MacFarlane, 2013),

> You feel like you're pulling teeth to get feedback. Even if I do a good job, there's something that I must need to improve

on, and so [when] the supervisors really don't give a lot of feedback . . . the feedback after sessions just takes longer to try and piece out exactly what went well from their perspective and what didn't go well. (p. 91)

As stated several times in this chapter, feedback should include sufficient positive and corrective comments: "Cultivating students' abilities to accurately self-assess both their strengths and growth areas by modeling balanced feedback is valuable for promoting self-reflective practice" (MacFarlane, 2013, p. 189). Research suggests genetic counseling students regard provision of balanced feedback as a positive supervisor skill (MacFarlane, 2013). Consider this student comment about supervisors who give mostly corrective feedback: "You're supposed to do the sandwich thing, you know, 'You did this well, here are 3 things to work on, and you did that well,' and sometimes it feels like the sandwich is just all meat and no bread" (MacFarlane, 2013, pp. 109–110).

No one ever conducts a perfect session, and no one totally ruins a session. Students will do some things that are skillful, and those behaviors should be encouraged. Acknowledging them in more than a token way is critical to increasing student self-awareness, confidence, and motivation to continue learning. Students will also do things that are less skillful and indicate the need for correction.

I suggest using what I call an *open-faced sandwich* approach in which the slice of bread (the foundation of the sandwich) is positive feedback, the filling is corrective feedback, and the toppings are ways to address the corrective feedback. An open-faced sandwich provides balanced feedback, reduces the pressure some supervisors feel to come up with another positive comment, and may seem less "gimmicky" compared to the traditional sandwich technique.

An elaborated version of this approach is the ask–tell–ask–teach feedback model (C. Peltier, personal communication, June

2, 2021), adapted from an ask–tell–ask model used with medical students (French et al., 2015). In the ask–tell–ask–teach model, the supervisor begins by requesting the student give specific examples of what went well. Then the supervisor responds with agreement and/or other skills the student did well. Next, the supervisor asks the student what did not go well or could have gone better. The supervisor again agrees and/or adds additional corrective feedback. The supervisor then provides either directive teaching about other ways to approach the problem or evocative teaching in which they invite the student's ideas followed by their own thoughts.

Example

> *Supervisor*: What do you think went particularly well in that session? (*Ask*)
>
> *Student*: I think I established rapport with the client and was able to provide her with the information she wanted about her test results.
>
> *Supervisor*: I agree, I think your explanations were very clear and I like that you checked in frequently to see what questions the client had. This allowed you to tailor your explanation to her needs. (*Tell*)
>
> *Student*: I've really been working on this, so it's good to hear it worked well.
>
> *Supervisor*: What aspect of the case do you feel didn't go as well as you would have liked? (*Ask*)
>
> *Student*: After explaining the results, the client seemed a little tearful. I'm glad you stepped in to ask how she was feeling because I didn't know what to say.
>
> *Supervisor*: Yes, I agree it was important to assess how she was feeling in addition to gauging her understanding. Let's talk about some questions you could ask to assess a client's feelings in a future session. (*Teach*)

Be Strategic, Selective, and Sensitive to Student Reactions

Genetic counseling student: I had someone who literally spent 40 minutes after every session, even if the session was only a 1/2-hour, talking about what I did well, what I did wrong . . . it was so draining!

—HENDRICKSON ET AL. (2002, P. 37)

When deciding how to approach feedback, ask yourself the following questions:

- Does it have to be said? (Choosing)
- Does it have to be said now? (Timing)
- Does it have to be said by me? (Directive or evocative)
- Does it have to be said this way? (Manner)

Feedback is an emotional process (Wherley et al., 2015). Expect some degree of defensiveness, especially when feedback is corrective and/or discrepant from a student's self-perceptions. In those situations, avoid getting into an argument. You will always have the final say, but when students publicly comply with what you want them to do, they may privately reject your feedback. I suggest saying something such as, "There are very few, if any, approaches that work equally well with every client. It's useful to develop a few different ways to go about things. Let's think about some additional strategies you can try for . . . ."

Provide Specific Feedback and Place It in a Context

Genetic counseling student: It's really hard to get negative feedback that's kind of vague to know how to improve from it, so I like really concrete feedback like, "You asked this question in this way, I think it would be better if you worded it differently like this," rather than saying, "You know, some of your questions . . . didn't work." I like

to know specifically what didn't work about them and how I can do
something different in the future to improve that.
—MACFARLANE (2013, PP. 106–107)

Telling a student "You did a good job" tells them nothing more than "You did not do a bad job." Telling a student "You did a bad job" does not tell them what a good job would be. Positive and corrective feedback are maximally helpful when stated as behaviorally as possible; include specific examples; and, in the case of corrective feedback, suggest an alternative approach.

Genetic counseling student: Hearing supervisors say that
everyone struggles with certain aspects of learning and genetic
counseling in general makes me feel better about any feelings of
inadequacy . . . [and] more confident in myself and my abilities by
them supporting and normalizing it for me.
—MACFARLANE ET AL. (2016, P. 760)

Whether giving a student positive or corrective feedback, provide guidance about its significance by connecting their behavior to its impact on the client or clients in general (e.g., how it made the client feel and the extent to which it helped or hindered the client's ability to understand and make a decision) and placing the student's behavior into a comparative frame (e.g., "This is challenging for most students at this point in their development," "Your skill at 'X' is at an advanced level," and "Being able to do 'X behavior' is a critical skill, so let's focus on that right now").

Recognize Corrective Feedback May Take Time to "Land"

When supervisors provide corrective feedback, they may fall into a trap of thinking, "Well, we discussed this a couple of times, and my student is still doing/not doing 'X' behavior." Then supervisors (and students) likely feel impatient and/or discouraged. I caution you against assuming your feedback did not "stick" when there is no visible behavior change. Genetic counseling skills are complex and require cognitive, affective, and behavioral changes. Consider the following suggestions:

- Remind yourself that incorporating feedback may be difficult and require multiple conversations and attempts. Students may be confused about what to do, how to do it, and/or when to do it. They may need time to internally process feedback and mentally rehearse before you will see behavioral changes.
- Discuss the student's internal processes: What does it mean if they are less than perfect? What are their feelings (e.g., fear, shame, and embarrassment)? What can they try next time?
- Work to identify smaller steps toward addressing the feedback (see mind mapping, Chapter 6).
- D. Langley (personal communication, January 8, 2010) recommends asking yourself these questions: What did I do today to help my student resolve corrective feedback? To what extent did I help my student clarify any misconceptions about the desired skill and associated behaviors? How do I know whether my student can apply behaviors related to the skill the next time they need to?

Provide Oral and Written Feedback

In addition to oral feedback, written feedback is helpful because it facilitates further student reflection at a later time. Written feedback is an "efficiently effective" method. For instance, it can help you recall and draw upon specific examples when engaging in feedback and when conducting mid-rotation and end-of-rotation evaluations. Asking students to take notes during debriefing meetings and sharing them with you provides one type of written material.

Supervisor note taking during genetic counseling sessions is another type of written material. A form may allow you to attend to student and client nonverbals and other aspects of counseling sessions more fully. If you take notes, I suggest sharing them with the student. Even if your handwriting is poor, they will be highly motivated to figure out what you wrote. Try to be discreet when taking notes (e.g., "Position yourself in the room to be out of the student and the client(s)' line of vision" [Hendrickson et al., 2002, p. 42]). You could develop a form to streamline note taking. Create a form that works for you and is comprehensible to the student. You might include the date and brief description of the session type (e.g., +trisomy results session). Some supervisors divide their note-taking page into four quadrants (positive feedback, corrective feedback, follow-up with client in session/after session, and miscellaneous). A follow-up quadrant may help minimize the number of step-ins you do in a counseling session.

Other supervisors list specific goals they wish to attend to in the session (e.g., Identified factors relevant to the client's decision-making), and they use a rating scale for each goal (1 = Not at all, 2 = Somewhat, 3 = Moderate extent, 4 = To a great extent). They also include space for a written comment (e.g., "You stated your understanding of the relevant factors clearly. Suggest you F/U with a question to see if the client agrees, such as, 'How does that sound to you?'").

Written feedback materials may also include a brief (5-minute) form that your student completes after each counseling session. Box 7.2 shows a form based on self-efficacy theory (Bandura, 1982).

BOX 7.2 Student Evaluation of Their Genetic Counseling

After the counseling session, complete the following:

Circle One:

0   1   2   3   4   5   6   7   8   9   10

My Worst Session   My Best Session

Why? (*1-2 sentences*):

My Degree of Certainty (*Circle One*):

0% 10% 20% 30% 40% 50% 60% 70% 80% 90% 100%

Students evaluate their counseling for each session by circling a number from 0 to 10 (where 0 = My worst session and 10 = My best session). Next, they briefly describe the reason for their rating. Then they circle a percentage from 0% to 100% to indicate their certainty about how well the session went.

You can also independently complete the form and use it to focus your feedback to the student. You can review the student's self-ratings daily or weekly, compare your ratings to those of the student, watch for expected improvement during the rotation, and intervene if necessary.

Written feedback methods have several benefits. They provide focus, promote feedback specificity, make your priorities and expectations explicit, provide data for formal evaluations (see Chapter 8), and comprise documentation in the event of problematic performance (see Chapter 13). Written feedback methods that involve student input provide a window into their priorities, concerns, and self-awareness.

Feedback Regarding the Supervisor and Supervision Relationship

No matter how good you think you are as a leader, my goodness, the people around you will have all kinds of ideas for how you can get better. So for me, the most fundamental thing about leadership is to have the humility to continue to get feedback and to try to get better—because your job is to try to help everybody else get better.
—JIM YONG KIM (AS CITED IN COGNOLOGY, N.D.)

Martin et al. (2014) recommend that

> supervisees and supervisors evaluate their sessions on a regular basis. Factors such as the style of supervision, whether the needs of the supervisee are being met, the effectiveness of feedback provided and the nature of the supervisory relationship, should be evaluated. (p. 205)

The strategies discussed here are intended to elicit feedback about yourself and the supervision relationship.

Supervisor Self-Feedback

Lehrman-Waterman and Ladany (2001) developed a scale for supervisees to evaluate supervisor goal setting and feedback skills. Eight items assess supervisor feedback skills (e.g., *My supervisor's comments about my work were understandable* and *My supervisor welcomed comments about his or her style as a supervisor*). You could evaluate yourself using the feedback items and corresponding rating scale and identify lower rated items as growth points.

Student Feedback

You could use items from Eubanks Higgins et al.'s (2013) supervisor competencies (see Chapter 1, Appendix 1A) to focus a conversation about the feedback process and other aspects of the supervision relationship at the rotation mid-point (or earlier). The Lehrman-Waterman and Ladany (2001) scale is also useful for inviting student comments about your feedback skills. If aspects of the feedback process could be improved, ask your student, "How could I/we do this better?" (Hendrickson et al., 2002, p. 42).

Chapter 6 contains a suggestion that supervisors ask students' programs to include the Lehrman-Waterman and Ladany (2001) goal-setting items when they collect end-of-rotation student evaluation data. They could include the feedback items as well.

Closing Thoughts

I believe *balance* is a useful overarching concept for approaching feedback. Feedback is more effective when it is the right amount (not too much or too little), focused (not too general or too picky), done sensitively (neither too harsh nor too mild), and a two-way process (not too much or too little from either the supervisor or the student). Perhaps most important, feedback should provide balanced support and challenge (neither predominantly positive nor predominantly corrective). I cannot stress enough the importance of encouragement along with correction when working with bright, engaged students. That sentiment is expressed in a quote from a psychotherapist working with a depressed client. The therapist asked her, "Why do you stand in the middle of the flowers and pick the weeds?" (Scraper, 2000, p. 14). Be sure to pay attention to the flowers along with the weeds when engaging in feedback with students.

Learning Activities

Most learning activities can be adapted for dyad or small group discussions or for written exercises. Time estimates are provided for discussions, but additional time should be allotted for large group processing.

Activity 7.1 Reflecting on Feedback

With a partner, discuss the following questions:

- How do you feel about giving positive feedback? Do you experience any challenges giving positive feedback?
- How do you feel receiving positive feedback? Do you experience any challenges receiving positive feedback?
- How you feel about giving corrective feedback? About receiving corrective feedback? What makes corrective feedback difficult for you to give and receive?
- Recall a time in your life when you received corrective feedback in a way that was hurtful/painful. How do you think that experience shapes what you do or will do when you give and receive feedback in the future?

Estimated time: 30 minutes

Adapted from McCarthy Veach, P., Willaert, R., & LeRoy, B. S. (2009). *Giving and receiving feedback in supervision: A DVD workbook*. University of Minnesota, Minneapolis, MN.

Activity 7.2 Feedback Challenges and Strategies

With a partner or in small groups, brainstorm responses to the following:

- What might supervisors do to sabotage feedback?
- What might students do to sabotage feedback?
- What can supervisors do to ensure feedback is balanced?
- What can supervisors do to ensure feedback has been communicated and understood?

Estimated time: 20 minutes

Note: This discussion can be expanded by asking participants to give an example of a time in supervision (either as a student or as a supervisor) when feedback was not understood, what contributed to the lack of understanding, and how the misunderstanding was rectified.

Adapted from McCarthy Veach, P., Willaert, R., & LeRoy, B. S. (2009). *Giving and receiving feedback in supervision: A DVD workbook*. University of Minnesota, Minneapolis, MN.

Activity 7.3 Challenging Student Responses to Feedback

With a partner or in small groups, identify possible reasons for each student statement and write a response. Write it as if you are speaking directly to the student:

You just don't like my style.
Motivation:
Your response:

Well, the client liked what I said.
Motivation:
Your response:

I don't know what you mean. I never did that.
Motivation:
Your response:

You didn't tell me I needed to prepare that information for the case.
Motivation:
Your response:

The reason I have trouble talking with clients is because you make me nervous.
Motivation:
Your response:

I really don't know what you want.
Motivation:
Your response:

Please don't tell the program director.
Motivation:
Your response:

Estimated time: 25 minutes

Adapted from McCarthy Veach, P., Willaert, R., & LeRoy, B. S. (2009). *Giving and receiving feedback in supervision: A DVD workbook.* University of Minnesota, Minneapolis, MN.

Activity 7.4 Challenging Supervisor Feedback Statements

With a partner or in small groups, identify what makes the supervisor's feedback challenging and rewrite the statement to make it more effective.

You did fine.
Challenging because:
Rewrite the statement:

You used the word "abnormal" to explain test results to the client.
   Never use that word.
Challenging because:
Rewrite the statement:

If you need any help, just let me know.
Challenging because:
Rewrite the statement:

[To a novice student after seeing their first client] *So, how do you*
   think that went?
Challenging because:
Rewrite the statement:

You should know this already.
Challenging because:
Rewrite the statement:

Well, it's not something I would have said to the client.
Challenging because:
Rewrite the statement:

The reason you're struggling is because you aren't trying hard enough.
Challenging because:
Rewrite the statement:

Estimated time: 25 minutes

Adapted from McCarthy Veach, P., Willaert, R., & LeRoy, B. S. (2009). *Giving and receiving feedback in supervision: A DVD workbook.* University of Minnesota, Minneapolis, MN.

Activity 7.5 Giving Feedback: Triad Role Plays

Take turns as supervisor, student, and observer for the following scenarios. After each role play, the student and observer should share their impressions of how the supervisor did identifying and addressing the issues requiring feedback.

- Student tells you they are personally against abortion and would rather not discuss it with a prenatal client unless the client brings it up first.
- After a session on BRCA risk assessment, the student says, "You did that whole session without ever referring to your notes. I don't think I could ever be as good as you."
- Student says, "But my other supervisor told me to record the family history the opposite way from what you're telling me to do."
- During the counseling session, the student reinforced the parents' mistaken belief that their child will grow out of phenylketonuria and can discontinue the diet as an adult. You are now debriefing the session.
- Your student comes to a debriefing meeting for a session that occurred yesterday and says, "I made a list of the things I said and did that were wrong—not as far as the information, but the way I said and did them. Here."
- Your student tells you at the beginning of the rotation that they think one of their strongest skills is building rapport with clients. After observing their interactions with several clients, you think the student needs to work on their rapport building (better eye contact, not interrupting the client, etc.).

Estimated time: 60–75 minutes

8

Evaluation in Supervision

CARRIE ATZINGER

Objectives

- Describe types and functions of student evaluation in supervision.
- Present approaches to student and supervisor evaluation.
- Discuss common challenges in evaluation and ways to manage them.
- Present strategies to promote an effective evaluation process.

Evaluation is the process by which supervisors determine and communicate whether a student has met expectations and is on track to successfully achieve competency as a genetic counselor by the end of their training. Ultimately, evaluation is critical to ensure that graduating professionals can provide high-quality care and services to genetic counseling clients (Bernard & Goodyear, 2014). Eubanks Higgins et al. (2013) outlined several genetic counseling supervisor competencies specific to evaluation (see Chapter 1, Appendix 1A). Box 8.1 lists these competencies.

> ### BOX 8.1 Genetic Counseling Supervisor Competencies—Evaluation
>
> - Specify and explain criteria used to determine if a student meets expectations set by the site and/or genetic counseling program.
> - Engage in active listening and observing during sessions.
> - Identify students' areas of strength and weakness.
> - Evaluate student performance and skill development for purposes of grade assignment or completion of a rotation.
> - Use evaluation tools to effectively document student skill development and progress during the course of the rotation.
> - Evaluate interpersonal dynamics among genetic counseling staff, other clinical and nonclinical personnel, patients, and students.
> - Collaborate with other genetic counseling colleagues also supervising the student if compiling a mid-point or final evaluation.
> - Provide a summative evaluation as a progress report to students midway through the rotation.
> - Provide a final summative evaluation which includes topics discussed in previous evaluations.
>
> ---
>
> *Source*: Eubanks Higgins, S., McCarthy Veach, P., MacFarlane, I. M., Borders, L. D., LeRoy, B. S., & Callanan, N. (2013). Genetic counseling supervisor competencies: Results of a Delphi study. *Journal of Genetic Counseling, 22,* 39–57.

Evaluation Functions and Criteria

Evaluation serves the primary function of assessing where a student stands in relation to expectations and/or specific criteria. Evaluation provides important information to the student and their graduate program faculty. In addition, the evaluation role (see Chapter 2) requires supervisors to act as gatekeepers preventing unqualified individuals from joining the field until they have reached standards of competence and professionalism (Bernard & Goodyear, 2014; McCarthy Veach & Leroy, 2009).

Formative Versus Summative Evaluation

When the cook tastes the soup, that's formative; when the guests taste the soup, that's summative.

—STAKE (1977, P. 169)

Formative evaluation involves ongoing assessment during a student's fieldwork rotation and often occurs through feedback interactions (see Chapter 7). Formative feedback provides an assessment of student progress toward goals established at the beginning of the rotation. Formative feedback is important in managing student anxiety related to evaluation by reducing the likelihood of an unexpected negative summative evaluation (MacFarlane et al., 2016).

Summative evaluation provides a big picture look at a student's strengths and growth areas; it is critical to student progress because it can inform goal setting and the strategies used in subsequent training experiences. Summative evaluation is more formal and focused on an overall assessment of a student's skills in relation to expectations appropriate to their point in training (Bernard & Goodyear, 2014; McCarthy Veach & LeRoy, 2009). Summative evaluations generally take place at the end of a rotation or at other set times, such as a rotation mid-point. Summative evaluations usually consist of two parts: verbal discussion with the student and written documentation for the student and their genetic counseling program to track progress over time (Bernard & Goodyear, 2014; McCarthy Veach & LeRoy, 2009).

Evaluation Criteria

Reflection Questions for Readers: Thinking about how you typically do evaluations in supervision (or imagining how you will do them), how do you know if a student is on track? What criteria do you use to assess their skills? How do you modify these criteria based on whether they are early or late in their training?

Many have noted that establishing evaluation criteria is the most difficult and crucial part of the evaluation process (e.g., Bernard & Goodyear, 2014). Generally, these criteria will involve a combination of specific knowledge, intervention skills, conceptualization skills, personalization skills, and/or professional behaviors (Bernard & Goodyear, 2014; see Chapter 6, this volume). Genetic counseling evaluation criteria typically align with the Accreditation Council for Genetic Counseling's (ACGC, 2019a) practice-based competencies (PBCs) regarding minimum knowledge and skills for an entry-level genetic counselor. Establishment of appropriate and clear criteria sets the stage for both formative and summative evaluation but does not dictate how the evaluation process occurs (Goodyear & Bernard, 2014).

Approaches to Student Evaluation

Currently, there are no standard evaluation instruments or scales used in genetic counseling training (Guy, 2016). Often, genetic counseling program leadership decides what evaluation scale(s) supervisors will use for their students. Consistency in evaluation scales across students' rotations is beneficial because it allows for comparison of evaluations and aids in tracking student progress over time.

Likert-Style Evaluations

A Likert-style evaluation form contains a standard scale to assess whether a student is meeting, exceeding, or falling below expectations for each performance criterion (Bernard & Goodyear, 2014). For example: "Presents information in an organized manner" [Scale: Meets expectations, Exceeds expectations, Falls below expectations, No basis for observation (NB)]. The following are additional examples of scales used in Likert-style evaluation forms: 1 = Poor, 2 = Below Average, 3 = Average, 4 = Above Average, 5 = Superior (numbers are not always included with these scale anchors); and Strongly Disagree, Disagree, Agree, Strongly Agree.

This type of assessment requires little training to complete, although it is highly susceptible to differences in supervisors' personal expectations (Bernard & Goodyear, 2014). If you use a Likert-style scale, it is important to orient the student to what behaviors align with ratings for each performance criterion, if they are not already defined. You should also have a conversation about what qualifies as a "good" or "passing" rating. A drawback of this type of scale is the limited number of rating choices. For instance, a student may receive "meets expectations" for a skill across every fieldwork experience because the expectations change across specialties and/or student developmental level. For this reason, a Likert-style scale does not easily show how a student is progressing in a skill over time.

Anchored Rubrics

Anchored rubrics are designed to highlight a student's progress over time by indicating the stage of development reflected in their performance of a particular skill (Bernard & Goodyear, 2014). Also referred to as competency-based assessment, anchored rubrics take a particular competency and break it into "levels"—for instance, *Functions at the level of a: Beginning rotation student, Mid-rotation student, Final rotation student, Practicing counselor*. Anchored rubrics tend to focus on outcomes and skill building. As described next, anchored rubrics may be generic, where every skill has the same rubric, or skill-specific, where each skill is broken into its own developmental levels (Bernard & Goodyear, 2014).

Generic Rubrics

Generic anchored rubrics use the same set of performance levels for each skill being assessed (Bernard & Goodyear, 2014), and each level should include a definition. Definitions may be based on how much supervision a student needs for each skill (e.g., *Functions extremely well and/or independently, Functions adequately and/or requires occasional supervision, Requires close supervision in this area, Not applicable to this training experience*), the level of complexity of the genetic counseling cases in which they are able to perform each skill, or frequency with which a student performs each skill at an acceptable level (e.g., *Never, Rarely, Sometimes, Often, Very often, Always*). Regardless of the definitions, a student's evaluations over time should show a progression from novice to independent for each skill (Guy, 2016). Importantly, variability in the complexity of different skills means students will be expected to progress at varying rates with different skills. In addition, prior experiences with the skills and opportunities to perform them mean individual students will progress at differential rates (Carraccio et al., 2008). Supervisors should normalize this variability with students. Generic anchored rubrics require that supervisors receive training on how to interpret the levels consistently to minimize bias and improve uniformity across fieldwork rotations (Carraccio et al., 2008).

The RIME framework is a generic rubric scale developed for use in medical education and employed by some genetic counseling programs. The RIME framework separates beginning and advanced stages of skill development using the terminology *Reporter–Interpreter–Manger–Educator* (Pangaro, 1999). RIME aims to incorporate assessment of many skills, knowledge, and attitudes (and their interactions) at each of four achievement levels (Pangaro, 1999). Reporting generally refers to "gathering and communicating clinical information" and demonstrating professionalism skills; interpreting is "reaching conclusions," such as generating differential diagnoses from information gathered; managing is "making plans" and tailoring interventions to client- and case-specific factors; and educating involves using metacognition about a skill to self-assess or be able to teach a skill to others (Pangaro & Cate, 2013, p. e1207). Progress through RIME levels is measured by the ability of students to perform skills at each level with increasing frequency. Because RIME is a developmental framework, typically students will achieve and maintain consistency in performing Reporter level skills before Interpreter level skills, and so forth.

Use of the RIME framework in genetic counseling evaluation requires clear definitions of what each level means for individual skills as set by a student's graduate program. Thus, clear definitions and training must be provided to supervisors, and supervisors should explain these definitions to students when using the RIME framework. Box 8.2 contains an example of RIME definitions for

---

BOX 8.2 Example of RIME Achievement Levels
for Interpersonal, Psychosocial, and Counseling
Skills Domain

Reporter: Describe genetic counseling process to clients. Elicit client expectations, perceptions, knowledge, and concerns regarding the genetic counseling encounter and the reason for referral or contact.

Interpreter: Apply client expectations, perceptions, knowledge, and concerns towards the development of a mutually agreed upon agenda.

Manager: Modify the genetic counseling agenda as appropriate by continually contracting to address emerging issues.

Evaluator: Identify how the genetic counselor's personal cultural characteristics and biases may impact encounters and use this knowledge to maintain effective client-focused services.

Source: Formal internship supervisor evaluation of student, Wayne State University Genetic Counseling Program, Center for Molecular Medicine and Genetics, Detroit, MI.

ACGC's (2019a) PBC Domain II: Interpersonal, Psychosocial, and Counseling Skills.

Another example of a generic rubric is based on the Dreyfus and Dreyfus model of skill acquisition (Carraccio et al., 2008). A student is evaluated on each skill as "Novice," "Advanced Beginner," "Competent," or "Proficient," as well as, in some instances, "Expert" or "Master." All students are expected to begin at a novice level and progress through different levels of development for every skill over the course of their training and, for some skills, throughout their career (Carraccio et al., 2008). Evaluation focuses on determining a student's level for each skill to provide them with the support they need to progress to the next level (Carraccio et al., 2008). In medical education, definitions of the skill levels have ranged from ability to apply a skill rigidly or flexibly in different situations, who is primarily responsible for a skill in a particular case, complexity of reasoning used to apply a skill, and commitment to ongoing skill improvement. These definitions leave a great deal of interpretation to individual supervisors (Carraccio et al., 2008).

Currently, no standardized definitions exist for applying rubrics based on RIME or the Dreyfus and Dreyfus model in genetic counseling supervision. Thus, as stated above, programs using these types of assessments must provide training for supervisors to ensure definitions are clear and to improve consistency. Training students in the definitions can also be helpful in establishing a shared language to use in supervision. Case-based examples can be a helpful training tool (Carraccio et al., 2008). As an individual supervisor, it is important to review the definitions of each level with a student to ensure you are on the same page regarding their meaning.

Skill-Specific Rubrics

Skill-specific rubrics contain scales that break development into a stepwise progression of achievements or "milestones" specific to each individual skill (Guy, 2016). Each scale outlines what

BOX 8.3 Example of a Skill-Specific Rubric for One
Practice-Based Competency

Practice-based competency: Establish a mutually agreed
upon genetic counseling agenda with the client.

Novice level: Student is able to identify and discuss with their
supervisor their goals before a session and the client's goals
after a session.

Advanced beginner level: Student is able to identify their goals
before a session and elicit the client's goals during the
session. Student is able to discuss with the client how goals
will be addressed in the session.

Competent level: Student is able to elicit a client's goals for a
session and establish an agenda that incorporates these
goals. Student discusses this agenda with the client and
modifies the agenda based on client's feedback.

Proficient level: Student is able to elicit a client's goals for a
session and discuss a mutual agenda for the session that
incorporates these goals. Student checks in with the client
throughout the session and modifies the agenda as needed
throughout the session. Student focuses on client agenda
rather than their own.

competency might look like at early and later stages of skill development and experience (Guy, 2016). Box 8.3 contains an example
of a skill-specific rubric for one genetic counseling PBC.

Although more time-consuming to develop, a skill-specific rubric may provide students with clearer explanations of what progression will look like for each skill (Bernard & Goodyear, 2014).
This type of rubric may also be easier for supervisors to use because developmental levels are defined. There are currently no
standardized milestones for genetic counseling skill development,
however (Guy, 2016).

Qualitative Feedback

No evaluation tool will be able to provide all necessary feedback to a student about their progression toward genetic counseling practitioner. Although feedback is covered in detail elsewhere (see Chapter 7), it is important to note that verbal and written feedback are a critical part of any evaluation. Supplementing numerical or categorical ratings with a qualitative narrative provides students (and their training programs) with information about why certain ratings were chosen and what observations were made to support these ratings. Both verbal and written feedback allow for interactive discussion with the student, and written feedback provides documentation for reference by program leadership and, in some cases, future supervisors. For students who ultimately cannot achieve competency, it is important to have clear and specific documentation of the fact (see Chapter 13).

Client Feedback

Another measure of student progress is the extent to which they successfully meet clients' needs (McCarthy Veach & LeRoy, 2009). One method for gaining input on a student's evaluation is to invite anonymous client feedback. If a clinic has an existing client feedback tool for its practitioners, it could be a mechanism for getting feedback about student performance. If not, you could, for instance, create a brief, two- or three-question feedback form and ask clients to complete it at the end of an encounter or at a later time (McCarthy Veach & LeRoy, 2009). You could also disseminate this form via email. Importantly, you should obtain approval from your clinic manager or institution for the form and process. In practice, this type of evaluation may be easier to implement in some rotation settings than others. A client feedback form may be a particularly useful tool in simulated or standardized patient scenarios in which there is less concern about the process causing undue burden to the client (for information on using standardized patients in supervision, see Chapter 15). You should always review client feedback with students and contextualize client comments because you have greater familiarity with expectations.

Student Self-Evaluation

Student self-evaluation is another important aspect of the evaluation process (Bernard & Goodyear, 2014; see also Chapter 7, this volume). Encouraging students to recognize and share perceptions of their skill development can promote self-reflective practice (Bernard & Goodyear, 2014; see also Chapter 9, this volume). In addition, it can allow supervisors to see how closely the student's perceptions match their own. Self-assessment may help supervisors anticipate students' reactions to evaluations and provide insight into how ready they are for independent practice. One approach to student self-evaluation is to have you and the student complete the same evaluation form separately and then discuss the ratings together. You could ask the student to complete the form twice—once the way *they* would evaluate themselves and once the way they think *you* will evaluate them. Discussion could then include noting areas of agreement and disagreement in the three sets of ratings.

Another source of information is to have students complete the Genetic Counseling Self-Efficacy Scale (GCSES) (Appendix 8A), which is a standardized scale for measuring self-efficacy for skills related to the PBCs (Caldwell et al., 2018a). Self-efficacy is an individual's perception of whether they can successfully perform a skill; and it has been shown to be related to whether they persevere when facing a challenging situation (Bandura, 1982). A student's self-efficacy ratings can provide information about the accuracy of their self-perceptions and help you determine skills for which they may need extra intervention. Asking the student to complete the scale at the beginning of the rotation, at mid-point, and at the end of the rotation can facilitate both formative and summative evaluation.

Evaluation Challenges

Any type of evaluation involves supervisor judgment of complex skills and, as such, poses challenges. Two prevalent challenges are subjectivity and power dynamics.

Subjectivity

No matter how objective we try to make an evaluation process, subjectivity is inevitable. Awareness of subjectivity pitfalls can help you manage and minimize these issues (Bernard & Goodyear, 2014). Evaluation measures are subject to response biases (e.g., the halo effect and generosity). Moreover, research has shown that supervisors may be impacted by how similar a student is to themselves. Perceived similarity generally results in higher ratings, but the opposite can also be true (e.g., a young supervisor may give a higher rating if a student is older) (Bernard & Goodyear, 2014). Stylistic differences may also result in lower ratings if a supervisor judges a skill as deficient when the student is just implementing it in a way that differs from that of the supervisor (Bernard & Goodyear, 2014). Knowing a student well through having worked with them in another role such as instructor or research advisor may also result in more (or less) favorable evaluations (Bernard & Goodyear, 2014).

Familiarity and similarity factors may be especially problematic because genetic counseling supervisors are predominantly White, cisgender, able-bodied women, which creates potential for bias in evaluations of those with underrepresented identities. Indeed, research has shown that some genetic counseling students believe they have received lower evaluations based on their gender or race (Aamodt et al., 2020). Training in implicit bias and implementation of mitigation strategies are key to minimizing real or perceived bias in evaluations (Mateo & Williams, 2020; see also Chapter 4, this volume). Including an implicit bias statement at the top of written evaluations can provide a reminder to supervisors to consider their predilections. The following is an example: "Evaluation involves a certain amount of subjectivity due to supervisor and student individual and cultural differences in values and perceptions. Approaching evaluation openly and thoughtfully and focusing on established goals and expectations can help to minimize implicit biases."

Power Dynamics

Supervisors inherently have power in supervision, and power differentials are especially apparent in the evaluation process. Ultimately, supervisors have the "final say" in providing an assessment of whether a student is meeting expectations, and this assessment has major consequences for the student (Bernard & Goodyear, 2014). This power imbalance means supervisors must take responsibility for establishing a trusting relationship and eliciting student reactions to feedback (Bernard & Goodyear, 2014). In addition, genetic counseling students have reported that the subjectivity and high-stakes nature of evaluation result in higher anxiety (MacFarlane et al., 2016). Giving frequent formative feedback throughout a rotation and providing specific examples during evaluations may help reduce student evaluation anxiety (MacFarlane et al., 2016).

Strategies for Promoting an Effective Evaluation Process

Several strategies can help create a positive environment for evaluation and help reduce student anxiety and defensiveness (Bernard & Goodyear, 2014; McCarthy Veach & LeRoy, 2009; MacFarlane et al., 2016):

- *Build a strong supervisory relationship.* Fostering a trusting, supportive relationship with the student helps reduce defensiveness. An important piece of this trust is setting and maintaining boundaries to avoid real or perceived conflicts of interest when conducting evaluations (see Chapter 11).

- *Be clear and specific.* Describe your role in evaluation (e.g., who assigns grades or determines whether a student "passes" a rotation). Provide feedback that is specific and supported by observations and examples to reduce ambiguity.
- *Incorporate multiple evaluation sources.* Data from sources such as supervisor assessment, student self-assessment, and client assessment (if feasible) will help reduce bias and validate feedback.
- *Encourage standardization.* The methods and timing of evaluation should be consistent across students whenever possible. Genetic counseling training programs often have their own evaluation forms to help with standardization of reporting.
- *Address student emotions.* Talk openly with students about how the evaluation process is impacting them. Let them know some anxiety and defensiveness are common reactions.
- *Be straightforward and consistent.* Strive for coherence in the feedback you give during the rotation and in your summative evaluations. Final feedback, in particular, should not "blind side" a student. Consider using language from formal evaluation scales to guide ongoing feedback conversations to help students "connect the dots" between formative and summative evaluations.
- *Have a clear administrative structure.* This is a shared responsibility with the program leadership. You should discuss with the student the evaluation process and what will happen after. How will the final feedback be documented and with whom will that documentation be shared? What will happen if a student does not meet expectations? If remediation is required, who will organize and evaluate this remediation (i.e., the supervisor or the program)? This conversation should begin at the outset of supervision and be reviewed as needed. If you are not familiar with program

processes, reach out to program leadership so that students get consistent messages.

Evaluating the Supervisor

For teachers, as for students, the most effective evaluation comes from someone who sits beside us and helps us grow.
— CAROL ANN TOMLINSON (2021, LAST PARA.)

Supervision is a skill to be developed and honed over time (Bernard & Goodyear, 2014; McCarthy Veach & LeRoy, 2009). Therefore, inviting summative evaluation from students about the supervision you provided can help you reflect on and improve your practice. As with student evaluation, supervisor evaluation can involve a variety of criteria and methods. Supervisors may ask students for verbal feedback on what went well and what could be improved. It is critical that this request occurs after the student's evaluation is finalized. Alternatively, students' graduate programs could ask them to provide anonymous feedback using a survey, or gather a combination of anonymous and direct feedback to promote both honest and immediate feedback. To preserve anonymity, programs could send collated feedback from several students. Although less immediate, this may still be useful feedback, especially if there is consistency across students.

Closing Thoughts

Evaluation is an essential and challenging component of supervision. Evaluation provides a big picture view of how a student is progressing in their skill development and serves the role of protecting clients. There are many methods and approaches to evaluation, but all require setting clear criteria and keeping evaluation methods consistent across students. The subjective nature of evaluation and the power dynamics within supervision mean that to be most effective, supervisors must create a strong supervisory relationship and work to minimize bias.

Learning Activities

Most learning activities can be adapted for dyad or small group discussions or for written exercises. Time estimates are provided for discussions, but additional time should be allotted for large group processing.

Activity 8.1 Summative Versus Formative Evaluation

Discuss these questions with a partner or in small groups:

- How are summative evaluations and formative evaluations (feedback) the same? Different?
- How do you/might you incorporate formative feedback into a final evaluation of a student?
- What challenges have you found to be specific to summative evaluation compared to formative evaluation?
- Think of your best summative evaluation experience (either as a supervisor or as a student). What made it the best? What about your least effective summative evaluation experience? What made it the least effective?

Estimated time: 20 minutes

Activity 8.2 Skill-Specific Anchored Rubrics

Working in small groups, for each of the following PBCs, describe what this skill should look like when performed by students who are at the following stages: novice, advanced beginner, competent, and proficient. [*Hint*: You may wish to refer to the example in Box 8.3.]

- Construct relevant, targeted, and comprehensive personal and family histories and pedigrees
- Promote client-centered, informed, noncoercive and value-based decision-making
- Effectively educate clients about a wide range of genetics and genomics information based on their needs, their characteristics, and the circumstances of the encounter
- Establish and maintain professional interdisciplinary relationships in both team and one-on-one settings and recognize one's role in the larger health care system

Estimated time: 45–60 minutes

Note: Each small group could be assigned one of the PBCs. The RIME Reporter, Interpreter, Manager, and Educator levels could be used instead for this activity.

Activity 8.3 Evaluating Student Goals

Students may begin a rotation with certain goals they would like to achieve. With a partner or in small groups, determine how you would evaluate student *progress* for each of the following goals. Begin by converting each goal to one that is specific and measurable (see Chapter 6).

- Improve my psychosocial assessment skills
- Get more experience with identifying and ordering genetic testing for clients
- Improve my ability to adjust my agenda to meet the client's goals
- Work on cancer risk assessment
- Incorporate questions to assess whether a client has religious or spiritual needs

Estimated time: 30 minutes

Activity 8.4 Qualitative Final Evaluation: Triad Role Plays

Take turns as supervisor, student, and observer for the following scenarios involving qualitative discussion of the final evaluation. After each role play, the student and observer should share their impressions of how subjectivity and power dynamics may have influenced the interaction.

Scenario: This is the student's first rotation. The student improved in their case preparation skills as well as their ability to take a family and medical history. The student needed considerable guidance for all other skills and has not yet begun to incorporate psychosocial assessment and counseling. This student has a lot of room for growth but is where you expect them to be at this point in their training.

Scenario: This is a student's second rotation in your specific specialty. The student performed all skills consistently for routine clients but had trouble adjusting if there was something complex or unexpected. Although this student is improving, you believe they may need more experience in this specialty to develop these more complex skills.

Scenario: This is the student's final rotation. The student is performing all skills at a level you would expect for a student getting ready to graduate. There are a couple of areas that you think the student will continue to improve as they get more experience after graduation, specifically discussing aspects of insurance coverage and privacy protections with clients. You want to discuss these areas for improvement while still reassuring the student they are meeting expectations.

Scenario: Your student completed the GCSES prior to meeting for their mid-rotation evaluation. You realize the student's ratings on many skills are higher than you would have expected based on their performance thus far. You are concerned the student is not able to self-assess their performance accurately. You want to discuss this concern while also reassuring the student that it is ok to still need to improve in skills at this point in their training.

Scenario: Client feedback for the student you are working with indicates the student builds strong rapport and clients feel supported. Several clients felt the information they received from the student was confusing. You want to incorporate this feedback into your evaluation of the student.

Estimated time: 45–60 minutes

Activity 8.5 Client Feedback Forms

Working in small groups (by specialty, if possible), develop a client feedback form and feedback process. Consider the following as you develop the form:

- What skill(s) or aspect(s) of the student's provision of genetic counseling would you like the client to assess? Does the client have the knowledge and information they need to provide a valid assessment?
- What type of scale will you use for this assessment (Likert scale, yes/no scale, etc.)?
- Will there be open-ended questions?
- How many questions are reasonable to ask a client to complete?
- How will you implement the collection of feedback using this form?

Estimated time: 20 minutes

Appendix 8A
Genetic Counseling Self-Efficacy Scale

*A number of competencies are described below that may be part of a genetic counseling session. Please rate how certain you are you can independently perform this competency **today** in a genetic counseling session.*

0   10   20   30   40   50   60   70   80   90   100

Not at all certain I can do   Moderately certain I can do   Highly certain I can do

1. Accurately record a family history by drawing a pedigree using appropriate pedigree symbols.
2. Formulate targeted, structured questions pertinent to an individual case in order to elicit a family history.
3. Ask targeted questions in order to elicit pertinent information from a client's medical history.
4. Assess the accuracy with which a diagnostic genetic/genomic test identifies a client's clinical status (clinical validity).
5. Assess the value of a diagnostic genetic/genomic test for determining treatment and management (clinical utility).
6. Select the most appropriate laboratory and genetic/genomic test for the given clinical situation.
7. Discuss potential benefits, risks, and limitations of genetic/genomic testing with a client.
8. Discuss potential costs of genetic/genomic testing with a client.
9. Facilitate the ordering of appropriate genetic/genomic testing for the client.
10. Interpret the clinical implications of genetic/genomic test reports.
11. Evaluate familial implications from genetic/genomic test results.
12. Incorporate the results of screening, testing, family history, environmental and lifestyle factors, and other relevant information to provide accurate risk assessment for clients (e.g., probability of carrier status, cancer risk assessment).
13. Modify the case management plan as needed in order to incorporate changes in management and surveillance recommendations.

14. Present the genetic counseling encounter information orally to other health care providers in a clear and concise manner (e.g., case presentation to physician).
15. Document the genetic counseling encounter information in accordance with professional guidelines and standards (e.g., medical record documentation; letters to other providers).
16. Identify appropriate resources, services and support for a client.
17. Establish a mutually agreed upon genetic counseling agenda with the client.
18. Explain the genetic counseling process to a client.
19. Contract with the client throughout the encounter to address emerging concerns.
20. Assess pertinent information relating to psychosocial history such as client emotions, individual and family experiences, beliefs, behaviors, values, coping mechanisms, and adaptive capabilities.
21. Respond with empathy to client's emotions and concerns.
22. Respond to a client's emotional and behavioral cues, expressed both verbally and nonverbally.
23. Respond to a client using normalization in a genetic counseling session.
24. Utilize anticipatory guidance in a genetic counseling session.
25. Utilize advanced empathy in a genetic counseling session.
26. Utilize in-depth exploration of client responses to risks and options.
27. Evaluate the need for intervention and referral for a client based on their psychosocial needs.
28. Implement evidence-based models of counseling to a genetic counseling session as appropriate (e.g., short-term client-centered counseling, grief counseling, crisis counseling).
29. Facilitate client decision-making that is consistent with the values of the client.
30. Maintain professional boundaries by ensuring directive statements, self-disclosure, and self-involving responses are in the best interest of the client.

31. Respond to client–counselor relationship dynamics, such as transference and countertransference.
32. Utilize an appropriate degree of directive or nondirective guidance for specific genetic counseling encounters.
33. Respond to client cultural beliefs relevant to the genetic counseling session.
34. Utilize risk communication principles and theory to maximize client understanding.
35. Communicate relevant genetic information to a client to help them better understand certain conditions.
36. Communicate with clients in a way that is clear and unambiguous based on the client's needs and circumstances of the encounter.
37. Present balanced descriptions of lived experiences of people with various conditions to a client.
38. Respond to ethical and moral dilemmas that may arise in genetic counseling practice.

Source: Caldwell, S., Wusik, K., He, H., Yager, G., & Atzinger, C. (2018a). Development and validation of the Genetic Counseling Self-Efficacy Scale (GCSES). *Journal of Genetic Counseling*, 27, 1248–1257. Reprinted with permission from the *Journal of Genetic Counseling*.

9

Supervision for Self-Reflective Practice

PATRICIA MCCARTHY VEACH

Objectives

- Define self-reflective practice.
- Describe self-reflection as a key component of deliberate practice.
- Present strategies for promoting student self-reflective practice.

Hindsight, if interpreted with care, is what brings us wisdom.
—WINSPEAR (2010, P. 239)

What Is Self-Reflective Practice?

Self-reflective practice is a deliberate process that "makes meaning from experience and transforms insights into practical strategies" (Chartered Institute of Personnel and Development [CIPD], n.d., p. 2). There are five components (p. 2):

- Learning to pay attention—listening to ourselves
- Coming face to face with our assumptions
- Noticing patterns
- Changing *what* we see
- Changing the *way* we see

Self-reflection is a key element of deliberate practice. It is a cognitive process in which a person critically evaluates their feelings, thoughts, and behaviors in each situation to produce insight and changes (Orchowski et al., 2010). Self-reflection involves four stages: "re-inhabit (relive the experience), reflect (notice what was going on), review (critically analyse the situation), reframe (capture new understanding)" (CIPD, n.d., p. 4).

When practitioners engage in self-reflection, their goal is "deliberate, active seeking of growth and development. . . .As such, reflection is not simply thinking, or ruminating without purpose" (Reiser, 2021, p. 351). Critically reflecting on experience allows practitioners to engage in continuous learning (Schon, 1991).

Self-reflection is necessary to meet Accreditation Council for Genetic Counseling (2019a) practice-based competencies such as seeking feedback and being responsive to performance evaluations, and it is necessary for ethical practice (Wherley et al., 2015). Research indicates genetic counselors learn from their professional experiences through periods of self-reflection (e.g., Miranda et al., 2016; Zahm et al., 2016). Self-reflection is a conduit for lifelong maintenance and enhancement of professional skills that are necessary for deliberate practice.

World renowned cellist Pablo Casals continued to practice 5 hours to 6 hours a day well into his 80's because as he once stated, "I think I am making progress."

—LEE (2016, P. 895)

Deliberate practice involves "individualized training activities . . . to improve specific aspects of an individual's performance through repetition and successive refinement" (Ericsson & Lehmann, 1996, pp. 278–279). Deliberate practice includes "mentally running through and reflecting on past and future [counseling] sessions" (Hill et al., 2017, p. 37).

Self-Reflection in Supervision

One of three outcome goals of the Reciprocal-Engagement Model of Supervision (see Chapter 1) states that the genetic counseling student "understands and applies information to engage in self-reflective practice" (Wherley et al., 2015, p. 715). Self-reflection is a central activity in clinical supervision (Borders, 2014; H. Holt et al., 2015; Martin et al., 2014), and it is part of genetic counselor supervisor competencies, namely to "encourage development of critical reasoning skills [and] promote student self-evaluation, self-exploration, and problem-solving abilities" (Eubanks Higgins et al., 2013, p. 55).

Supervision is an ideal environment for the intentional cultivation of self-reflective skills because students are not only encouraged to discuss their genetic counseling experiences but also have the opportunity to consider them with support from more experienced practitioners. The supervisor and student work to understand the student's internal responses (feelings and thoughts) and how the student makes meaning of events eliciting those responses (Orchowski et al., 2010). The results of their efforts "may include new knowledge or specific adjustments" to their behavior (Orchowski et al., 2010, p. 52). Supervisors foster self-reflective practice through evocative processes (e.g., those described in this chapter) that guide students to critically analyze their work and modify their approaches as needed (Wherley et al., 2015). At the highest skill level, "students are able to reflect on session dynamics as they occur and adjust their counseling accordingly" (Wherley et al., 2015, p. 715).

Strategies for Promoting Student Self-Reflective Practice

A variety of strategies can infuse student self-reflection within supervision. Strategies range from setting expectations for self-reflection to building students' self-reflective skills throughout a rotation. Importantly, these strategies have maximal effects when "captured and expressed in some form—usually written, spoken or pictorial—on a systematic basis. This is because learning comes not only from the 'in the head' reflection but from the process of representing the reflection itself" (CIPD, n.d., p. 3). Several strategies are described next.

Cultivate and Model Your Own Self-Reflection Skills

Cultivation

Student reflection starts with the supervisor's reflective process (Orchowski et al., 2010). Aim to remain open and responsive to feedback, willingly admit you are less than perfect, and view your genetic counseling and supervision skills as a lifelong "work in progress." In addition, approach your self-reflective practice with confidence and engage in ongoing self-assessment of your professional activities. These efforts will enhance your self-reflection skills, which in turn will aid you in encouraging student self-reflection efforts.

Modeling

Modeling self-reflective practice is a powerful strategy for promoting student self-reflection (Orchowski et al., 2010). Modeling will occur in all supervision activities: case preparation when you give your perspective about an upcoming case; sessions in which your student observes you counseling a client and then when you share thoughts and feelings you had as you counseled; debriefing when you reflect on and then share the internal reactions you experienced as your student counseled a client; and discussions in which you share your thoughts and feelings about the supervision relationship, your student's professional development, and so forth. Self-reflective practice can be helpful for a variety of issues, such as considering puzzling situations, generating hypotheses about underlying dynamics, and exploring how to proceed in the future. When you model "the process of 'looking inward' . . .[you] can communicate the importance of understanding the processes by which individuals construct meaning from events, which may ultimately result in a deeper understanding of how individuals function together" (Orchowski et al., 2010, p. 55).

Set the Stage with Directed Self-Reflection Protocols

Establish an expectancy at the beginning of supervision that the student will engage in self-reflection about their genetic counseling practice as well as their supervision experiences. One strategy for beginning the process is to use directed self-reflection protocols before your first supervision meeting. Moffett (2009) created the directed self-reflection protocol as a supplemental method to help novice supervisees anticipate working with unfamiliar client populations, service delivery models, and/or practice settings. The protocol consists of a series of questions to elicit supervisee self-reflection about their impending work. Moffett asserts that self-directed protocols help build empathy and allow supervisees to anticipate their possible thoughts, feelings, and behaviors in clinical situations.

To use this strategy, begin by developing a list of questions about issues that tend to be challenging at your practice site. Prior to starting the rotation, give the list of questions to the students. Ask them to reflect upon the questions and privately write answers as a way of priming themselves for potential challenges. Questions should ask about concrete reactions in potential situations (e.g., Under what conditions would you . . .? What would you think when . . .? What would you feel when . . .? What would you do when . . .?). Importantly, you *should not* ask students to share their answers with you. Private self-reflection will "promote more thorough and honest deliberations by reducing the anxiety of being evaluated and the pressure to give conventional answers" (Moffett, 2009, p. 79). Students, however, will often voluntarily share (to differing extents) aspects of their answers as specific issues arise in clinic.

The types of questions you can ask are virtually limitless. Furthermore, questions can pertain to the student's clinical work as well as their supervision relationship with you. Box 9.1

BOX 9.1 Examples of Directed Self-Reflection Protocol Questions for Students

Questions About Clinical Work

- What do you think when your efforts to help someone do not work?
- What do you feel when your efforts to help someone do not work?
- What do you do when your efforts to help someone do not work?
- What do you want from persons you try to help?
- What are acceptable ways for someone to express anger toward you?
- What do you do when someone you are attempting to help doesn't listen to you?
- How do you decide whether to answer a client's personal questions?
- How do you know if you have helped a client?
- What do you do when clients ask about a condition you did not prep for?

Questions About Supervision

- What sorts of things could you do to feel at ease in supervision?
- What sorts of things might I do to help you feel at ease?
- How might we handle differences of opinion?
- What fears do you have regarding feedback?
- What do you hope I will say about you at the end of the supervision rotation?

contains several examples of broad questions for students to reflect on regarding their clinical work and supervision. These questions can also be useful as the basis for classroom discussion. Of note, protocols for a given setting typically will include questions that are more specific (e.g., How will you feel counseling a family whose child has just died?).

Here are some suggested steps for using a self-directed protocol with students: Explain its purpose; reassure your student that you will not ask to see their answers; if questions are quite challenging, give them a few at a time (to avoid overwhelming students); and include questions about gratifying aspects of the rotation (e.g., What do you think will be the most rewarding part of this rotation? How will you feel when a client says you were helpful?).

A directed self-reflection protocol can also help promote your own contemplation about starting supervision with a student. Box 9.2 contains examples of questions you could ask yourself.

Additional Benefits of Self-Directed Protocols

Moffett (2009) describes several benefits of self-directed protocols for supervisees. They accelerate the supervision process by making more concrete the types of fieldwork and supervisory experiences students are likely to have, suggest that any topic is welcome for discussion without pressure to disclose beyond a student's comfort level, and help students recognize discrepancies between their predictions and their actual experiences and actions during their fieldwork. Moffett also notes that the process of creating a self-directed protocol for supervisees may help supervisors "clarify and sharpen their own understanding of the clinical endeavor" (p. 83). I believe additional benefits derive from protocols containing questions specific to a given setting. Specific questions provide students with a nuanced "orientation" to what it will be like to be in the rotation, and they direct student attention to experiences that may be the focus of their clinical and supervision work.

BOX 9.2 Examples of Directed Self-Reflection Protocol Questions for Supervisors

- Given any information I might already have about this student (e.g., from instructing them in a course, serving on their master's committee, or responses to "getting acquainted" questions I sent them [see Chapter 3]), what do I think I will find rewarding in working with them?
- What may be challenging in my supervision of this student?
- What is my biggest hope about working with this student?
- What is my biggest fear about working with this student?
- How do I feel about beginning a(nother) supervision relationship?
- How do I think these feelings will affect what I say and do in supervision?
- What did I learn from my last supervision relationship that I can apply to this one?
- How do I plan to handle conflicts that may arise between us?
- How am I usually (or how will I be) most helpful to the students I supervise?
- What do I hope this student will say about their supervision experience with me after the rotation?

I also believe self-directed protocols for supervisors yield similar benefits. They help concretize what the work of supervision may be like with a particular student, allow supervisors to take stock of their thoughts and feelings about beginning a supervision relationship, and aid supervisors in anticipating possible rewards and challenges.

Work on Minimizing Barriers to Student Reflective Practice

The *power differential* between supervisors and students is a common barrier to self-reflective practice because it makes some students hesitant to share their uncertainties (Orchowski et al., 2010). Building a strong working alliance (see Chapter 3) and cultivating and modeling self-reflective practice, as described previously, may help minimize this barrier.

Another prevalent barrier is the variability in *students' skill level* for engaging in reflective thinking (Martin et al., 2014). Novice students, in particular, may have limited experience with this skill, especially as it applies to a genetic counseling setting. Therefore, it is important to provide ongoing direction and support for their self-reflection attempts to reduce frustration and encourage skill building (Martin et al., 2014).

A third potential barrier is underestimating the amount of *anxiety* students have about clinical supervision (Orchowski et al., 2010; see also Chapter 14, this volume). Their anxiety may lead to excessive rumination; self-critical thinking; and defensiveness about supervisor feedback. Anxiety also causes some students to engage in impression management, and to routinely ask supervisors to "tell them what to do." Self-reflection should be about problem-solving and professional development rather than self-flagellation and self-protectiveness. Try to recognize these tendencies and work to help students gradually adopt a more engaged and balanced perspective. Focus discussion on how what they learn through self-reflection will enhance their future behavior.

The following hypothetical example describes a supervisor's responses (and their intended effects) when addressing an anxious student's extreme rumination (adapted from McCarthy Veach et al., 2009):

> *Scenario*: The student and supervisor are discussing how they handled a difficult cystic fibrosis newborn screen. The student was visibly nervous during the session and had difficulty providing the couple with the information they were requesting. The student has been having trouble maintaining self-confidence during counseling sessions in general.

Student: I was really nervous during that session and I think I did a pretty horrible job.

Supervisor: What made you so nervous? (*Evidence gathering*)

Student: The case was really complicated, and I didn't do a good job explaining things. The couple probably left more confused than when they came in.

Supervisor: You've done newborn screens before. What made you so nervous this time? (*Stimulus discrimination*)

Student: I think I was nervous because the parents seemed more visibly upset than other clients I've seen. They were worried, and it made me worried.

Supervisor: What do you think you could have done differently then? (*Reflect on behaviors the student could try in the future*)

Student: [Sighs] I don't know. . . . I still think it didn't go well. I made a list of all the bad things I did.

Supervisor: Only negative things? Did you list anything positive? Because I definitely think there are things you did well (*Avoids doing the self-reflective work for the student; shifts student thinking away from rumination to constructive self-reflection*)

Student: I can't think of anything that went very positively, only things I did poorly like confusing the couple and making them late for their next appointment.

Supervisor: I'm noticing a common theme here. We've done about 10 cases together, and usually you have a list of only things that did not go well. . . . Let's find a way for you to think about what you did well. Part of evaluating is thinking about how the whole case went, things you did well and want to continue doing and things you could consider doing differently. But it's nothing to beat yourself up over. (*Encourages a balanced self-appraisal*)

Student: I'm afraid of saying something wrong in sessions and messing up the clients' medical care. And when I can't answer every question, I feel like I'm not giving them the best service.

Supervisor: You put a lot of pressure on yourself. I can see that this is not just about this case but also about how you're doing overall. Is that right? (*Points out a pattern of self-defeating thoughts*)
Student: Yes.
Supervisor: Can you think of what went well that you did right in this counseling session? (*Turns focus from self-defeating thoughts to constructive self-reflection*)
Student: I can't think of anything [Pause]. . . . but I can think of something that went well in the case before this one.
Supervisor: Let's talk about that case. (*Reinforces student attempt to find evidence that disputes their "Everything I do is wrong" belief*)
Student: I think I established rapport and I was comfortable speaking with the couple.
Supervisor: I think you really connected with that family . . . they were in a lot of distress, and you did a great job calming them and letting them know it was okay to be worried. (*Reinforces constructive self-reflection*)
Student: The more I think about the current case, I guess the parents did seem less stressed when they left, so maybe I did give them some good information.
Supervisor: That's true, and it's not something to just brush away . . . you did help them. And if you think about your preparation for the case and the session itself, it's not one thing, but many things you did right. . . . We can talk more about those good things right now or next week. (*Reinforces and continues to shape student thinking toward balanced self-reflection*)
Student: Ok. I'll think some more about the positive things for when we talk next week.
Supervisor: Now, I don't want to discount your list. So, let's talk also about the things you want to do better. (*Conveys respect for and openness to the student's feelings and thoughts about their performance*)

Use Evocative Strategies

His questions had helped break down a wall so that she could see
a door ... the knowledge she had in the palm of her hand had been
there all the time. It had just taken a conversation ... to enable her
to recognize it.

—WINSPEAR (2010, P. 122)

Evocative strategies provide the space for self-reflection that helps students "identify lessons learned" from their experiences (Reiser, 2021, p. 351). Evocative strategies include "open-ended and non-judgmental questions, which are aimed at cultivating a deeper understanding" and help balance discussion of technical aspects of genetic counseling with the student's decisions about how they approached the session (Orchowski et al., 2010, p. 58).

You can encourage students to "think aloud" about questions such as the following: "What made the situation difficult? How did I respond and why? Is there anything I could do differently the next time I encounter a similar situation?" (Reiser, 2021, pp. 350–351). The following example illustrates a supervisor's evocative approach:

> *Student*: When the patient said their father just died of Huntington's disease and then began to cry and said they wanted to die, too, I didn't know what to say.
> *Supervisor*: How were you feeling when they said that?
> *Student*: Uncomfortable.
> *Supervisor*: What were you thinking about what they said?
> *Student*: I was trying to come up with something to make them feel better.
> *Supervisor*: What do you remember doing at that point?
> *Student*: I think I said I was sorry, and then I told them there's a test for Huntington's.
> *Supervisor*: You clearly felt compassion for them, which is a real strength. [Pause] Let's talk about what you think the patient needed in that moment and different ways you might have addressed their needs.

[Student and supervisor discuss alternative responses.]
Supervisor: What do you think you will do the next time something like this happens?

Give Students Self-Reflection Assignments to Complete Outside of Supervision Meetings
Case Preparation

Case preparation is an expected part of planning genetic counseling sessions. Typical topics for students to address include the following (Uhlmann, 2009): expected reasons a patient is seeking genetic counseling and possible patient questions; biomedical information, relevant research, and risk statistics given what is known about the patient and family history prior to the session; additional patient/family history to be gathered during the session; testing options, including their availability and utility; potential resources (support groups, publications, etc.); and visual aids if appropriate. Discussion of their case preps during supervision will help students assess the extent to which the content is relevant, accurate, and organized. Discussion will also help them reflect on how they will organize the topics during actual sessions (Uhlmann, 2009). Case preparation can also include anticipation of psychosocial issues that might arise during the session and how these might be managed.

Case Debriefing

Ask students to complete a checklist or a brief self-evaluation form (see Chapter 7) after sessions and prior to beginning debriefing meetings. Use this form to focus discussion of each counseling session.

Journaling

Journaling allows students to engage in a deeper level of processing than usually occurs "in the moment" of a supervision meeting (Orchowski et al., 2010) or other type of professional experience

(Reiser, 2021). Journaling can be either written or audio recorded. I recommend providing students with an overall structure for journaling. For instance, ask them to briefly describe the experience (remind them not to include identifying information about clients); what they felt, thought, and did; how the experience will affect what they do in the future; and unresolved aspects of the experience they wish to discuss with you. Decide whether you will review their journal entries or allow them to determine which content to share with you.

Debrief Role Plays and Counseling Sessions Using Interpersonal Process Recall

Interpersonal process recall (IPR) is a method designed to reflect systematically about videotaped counseling sessions (Kagan & Schauble, 1969). The supervisor and student view the tape together, and as they do so, either person can pause the tape to discuss relevant events in the session. Systematic questions facilitate discussion and include, for example, the following (Kagan, 1971; Miller et al., 1975):

- What did you do (i.e., present action)?
- What data from the client (verbal? nonverbal?) was your reaction based on?
- What were you thinking?
- What were you feeling? What physical sensations in yourself were you aware of?
- When else in your interactions with clients have you felt that way?
- What did you do in those situations (i.e., past action)?
- What impact did your actions seem to have on the client?

Because recordings of actual genetic counseling sessions are uncommon, the IPR method is most suitable for role play or standardized patient interactions. Nevertheless, a modified form of IPR can be effective for encouraging reflection about actual sessions. During live observation, write down one or two relevant segments. The segments can be about anything you believe is important to discuss (e.g., something the student did that was helpful or something the student did that was unhelpful). Briefly describe the context (explanation of testing options; "Pt said . . ., You said . . ."). During debriefing, use your notes about the segment to jog the student's memory and then discuss using IPR questions. You might also ask the student to identify one or two segments of the session they wish to talk about and structure that discussion using IPR questions. Given time constraints, it is a good idea to limit discussion to the most pivotal portions of a counseling session.

Use Processes from Socratic Dialogue During Supervision

Socratic dialogue is another evocative strategy for helping students engage in self-reflection. Socratic dialogue involves asking a series of questions to determine a supervisee's thoughts, feelings, and behaviors about a situation. Three Socratic dialogue processes, as described by Overholser (2004), are particularly relevant for genetic counseling: systematic questioning, inductive reasoning, and disavowal of knowledge.

Systematic Questioning

During case preparations, you can use systematic questions to help students anticipate and logically plan sessions, including session goals, priorities regarding session content, and counseling approaches. During session debriefings, you can use systematic questioning to help students evaluate their actual behaviors against their planned approach.

Examples of systematic case preparation questions, modified from Overholser (2004), are What do you think the client hopes to gain from the session? How realistic are those goals? and How might you help the client achieve those goals?

Examples of debriefing questions include What do you think the client hoped to gain from the session? How realistic were their goals? What did you do to help the client modify their goals or achieve the goals? and How effective do you think your approach was? Note that these questions ask students to compare their expectations of the session (case preparation) to what actually transpired.

Translation questions are a particular type of systematic questions intended to help students consider their fieldwork from different perspectives. Translation questions ask them to identify multiple ideas during case preparation and debriefing. For example, when a student tells you what they think client goals will be or what dynamics they noticed in a session, you can ask them to come up with at least one additional hypothesis. Translation questions help prevent students (and supervisors) from jumping to premature and perhaps inaccurate conclusions and from introducing unintended bias into their counseling and supervision work.

Inductive Reasoning

Inductive reasoning is a logical thinking process that involves combining existing knowledge, observations, and experiences to reach a conclusion (Overholser, 2004). Table 9.1 contains examples of questions that promote inductive reasoning.

Disavowal of Knowledge

Socratic dialogue also involves the supervisor engaging in "disavowal of knowledge"—that is, being open and honest about the fact that they are not always correct (Overholser, 2004). Importantly, you should approach the dialogue in a collaborative manner and acknowledge you do not have all the answers but that you and your student will figure it out together as you proceed.

TABLE 9.1 Examples of Questions to Encourage Inductive Reasoning

Clarification	What do you mean when you say . . .? Could you explain that further? Can you provide an example?
Challenging assumptions	What would be a different way of thinking about that? What assumptions might you be holding about . . .?
Evidence and reasoning	Can you provide an example that supports what you are saying? Can we validate that evidence? Do we have all the information we need?
Alternative viewpoints	Are there alternative viewpoints? How could a different person respond, and why?
Implications and consequences	How would this affect the client? What are the long-term implications of this?
Challenging the question	What do you think was important about this issue we discussed? What "takeaways" do you have from this discussion?

Adapted from Sutton, J. (2020). *Socratic questioning in psychology: Examples and techniques.* https://positivepsychology.com/socratic-questioning.

Tips for Using Socratic Dialogue

The following approaches to Socratic dialogue (adapted from Sutton, 2020, Guidance section) can facilitate the process: Plan significant questions to inform an overall structure and direction without being too prescriptive, stimulate the discussion with probing questions that follow the responses given, keep the dialogue focused and specific, regularly summarize the discussion, and reword questions that are vague and/or beyond the student's understanding. Importantly, systematic questions "should derive from a sincere search for information, and should not appear similar to an oral examination" (Overholser, 2004, p. 8). Keeping your questions as open-ended as possible will help prevent the dialogue from turning into a "cross-examination" and maximize the student's ability to consider multiple perspectives.

Closing Thoughts

When you provide students with opportunities for self-reflection, you plant the seeds for lifelong deliberate practice. Self-reflection is not an easily developed skill. It requires patience and effort on both the student's part and your part. For instance, usually you will be more confident than your student about your assessment of a client's needs and how to address them. Therefore, "it is easy to become dogmatic and simply tell the supervisee what to do" (Overholser, 2004, p. 10) or give a "quick fix" because you see your student struggling to figure out something. There are, of course, situations in which directiveness is necessary, but if you routinely take a directive approach, you will deny students the opportunity for growth (Overholser, 2004). As one genetic counselor shared about their experience supervising students, "One thing that's really hard is just keeping my mouth shut. I get very impatient when students struggle. . . .To just sit there, I can't tell you how much I squeeze my pen or pinch my leg just to bear it!" (Hendrickson et al., 2002, p. 37). So, squeeze your pen, pinch your leg, or take a deep breath, and see where your students go in their efforts to reflect and respond. And trust that although you may not have the "first word" when reflecting, you can always have the final word.

Learning Activities

Most learning activities can be adapted for dyad or small group discussions or for written exercises. Time estimates are provided for discussions, but additional time should be allotted for large group processing.

Activity 9.1 Creating a Self-Directed Protocol

We commonly fail to consider the reality of new situations or experiences. We also often imagine things that are *not* the other person's experience (differences in age, gender, culture, life experience, etc.). *Example*: Thinking all individuals would be devastated to have a baby with Down syndrome. With those points in mind, in small groups, do the following:

- Generate 10–12 questions you could ask a student to reflect upon before counseling clients at your site (example: "If you tested positive for spinocerebellar ataxia, what would you think about yourself? Feel? Who would you tell?").
- Generate 5–7 questions you could ask a student to reflect upon prior to starting a supervision relationship with you.

Estimated time: 40 minutes

Note: This activity works well when groups are formed based on practice specialty. In processing this activity, point out themes in the groups' protocols (some are more focused on student feelings and thoughts, some on their behaviors, etc.).

Adapted from Moffett, L. (2009). Directed self-reflection protocols in supervision. *Training and Education in Professional Psychology*, *3*, 78–83.

Activity 9.2 Engaging in Socratic Dialogue

Without giving any information that might identify the other individual, describe a supervision interaction in which a student (if you are a supervisor) or a supervisor (if you have not yet been a supervisor) said something that was puzzling/challenging to you. Then prepare a written response to the following inductive reasoning questions to reflect upon the situation. Share your responses with a partner.

Clarification: What was the situation? What did the other person say and do? What did you say and do?

Challenging assumptions: How did you explain the incident to yourself at the time? What would be a different way of thinking about that?

Implications and consequences: How did this incident affect you? What have been the long-term implications?

Challenging the question: What do you think was important about this incident? What "takeaways" do you have from reflecting on it now?

Estimated time: 30 minutes

Note: This exercise could be used to consider a situation with a client.

Activity 9.3 Supervision Self-Reflection

Identify *one* personal goal or aspiration for your further development of a supervision skill that you would like to achieve over the next 3 or 4 years.

- Create a mind map of your goal (described in Chapter 6).
  - Write the goal in the center of your paper.
  - Draw spokes around the goal.
  - List one step at the end of each spoke for achieving your goal.
- Share your mind map with a partner.
- Personally commit to taking these steps.

Estimated time: 25 minutes

Activity 9.4 Interpersonal Process Recall Debriefing: Role Plays

Record part of a standardized patient session or genetic counseling role play in which you are the counselor. Then with a partner, review each other's recordings using IPR questions listed in this chapter to debrief the session.

Estimated time: If the recording is done in advance, IPR debriefing of a partial session would be 20 minutes per recording.

Note: Supervisors can use this activity with their students who can role-play a partial session or a full session.

Activity 9.5 Using Evocative Strategies in Supervision: Triad Role Plays

Take turns as supervisor, student, and observer for the following scenarios. Use evocative strategies to address the issues in each scenario. After each role play, the student and observer should share their impressions of how the supervisor did addressing the issues with evocative strategies.

Scenario 1: Your supervisee, a novice genetic counseling student, asks you a lot of questions and solicits a lot of advice about how to proceed with clients. At the same time, however, they seem to deflect your suggestions. They have a "yes, but . . ." style of responding to your feedback.

Scenario 2: You are supervising a student who has a "know it all" attitude and is a little too overly confident for their level of experience. The student is resistant to feedback or suggestions. They will never admit that they do not know something even when it is obvious they are inadequately informed.

Scenario 3: Your student was independently counseling a couple for a portion of a session regarding the results of their son's testing for phenylketonuria (PKU). Although your student was prepared to counsel this case (based on your discussion with the student prior to the counseling session), they were unable to answer several basic questions the family had about PKU. The student ended up leaving the room to get you, and you had to "step in" to finish the session.

Estimated time: 45 minutes

10

Fostering Psychosocial Skill Development

PATRICIA MCCARTHY VEACH

Objectives

- Define psychosocial skills in genetic counseling.
- Discuss the importance of psychosocial skills in genetic counseling practice.
- Describe types of psychosocial skills critical to genetic counseling practice.
- Identify supervision strategies to foster student development of psychosocial skills.

What Are Psychosocial Skills and Why Are They Important?

It was when I recognized that my empathic attunement with patients and families brought the science to life that I really understood the genetic counseling experience.
—DJURDJINOVIC (2009, P. 133)

Reflection Question for Readers: When you hear the term psychosocial skills, what comes to mind?

The term *psychosocial skills* has meaning for every genetic counselor and genetic counseling student, although the nature of that meaning differs substantially across individuals. Moreover, the way a person defines the term plays a significant role in the extent to which they prioritize and approach psychosocial skills in their practice. *Psychosocial* refers to "having both psychological and social parts" (*Cambridge Dictionary*, 2021). Regarding psychosocial skills in genetic counseling, some authors describe them as distinct basic responses, such as questions, reflections of feeling, and nonverbal reactions, and as "skills for dealing with contextual (e.g., multicultural awareness) and situational (e.g., client resistance) concerns" (Borders et al., 2006, p. 212). Others describe psychosocial skills as "interventions that provide psychologically based discussions of genetic concerns . . . [the] interweaving of sociocultural strata with the psychological allows the genetic counselor to consider the counselee in his or her fullest complexity" (Djurdjinovic, 2009, p. 134).

The Accreditation Council for Genetic Counseling (2019a, p. 2) practice-based competencies include a domain of interpersonal, psychosocial, and counseling skills. Four categories within this domain include the following competencies:

- Establishing a mutually agreed-upon genetic counseling agenda with the client
- Employing active listening and interviewing skills to identify, assess, and empathically respond to stated and emerging concerns
- Using a range of genetic counseling skills and models to facilitate informed decision-making and adaptation to genetic risks or conditions
- Promoting client-centered, informed, noncoercive, and value-based decision-making
- Understanding how to adapt genetic counseling skills for varied service delivery models

- Applying genetic counseling skills in a culturally responsive and respectful manner to all clients

Eubanks Higgins et al. (2013; see also Chapter 1, Appendix 1A) identified several genetic counseling supervisor competencies related to building student psychosocial skills, including the following:

- Encourage development of critical reasoning skills
- Require students to consider relevant ethical issues and cultural considerations in planning for sessions
- Assist students in incorporating patient psychological and behavioral characteristics into the genetic counseling session
- Assist students in adjusting counseling goals for a patient based on ongoing assessment and evaluation during the genetic counseling session
- Guide and evaluate students' abilities to permit the patient to express intense emotional states and help students manage extreme patient behaviors
- Elicit students' perceptions of patient psychosocial dynamics
- Help students process and learn effective coping strategies for emotionally difficult cases

Psychosocial skills are critical for helping genetic counseling clients reflect on their thoughts and feelings related to making decisions, managing their condition, and adapting to their situation (McCarthy Veach et al. 2007; Shugar, 2017). Client emotions are especially important because, as McCarthy Veach et al. (2007) note, they

interact with all facets of genetic counseling processes and outcomes, for instance, affecting their desire for information, their comprehension of information, the impact of information on their decisions, their willingness and ability to connect with the counselor, their desire for autonomy, and their perceived resilience. (p. 722)

As Seymour Kessler (2000) cautions,

having and expressing emotion are normal human reactions to joy, disappointment, pain, loss, failure, bereavement, and so on. . . . Some professionals seem to view emotions through a lens of pathology; such reactions ought to be avoided and suppressed . . . this is unfortunate since what most people want when they are in distress is understanding, empathy, and comforting." (p. 276)

Types of Psychosocial Skills

Psychosocial skills are complex and multidimensional. Bernard's Discrimination Model (Bernard, 1979, 1997; see also Chapter 6, this volume) is useful for considering these types of skills. Bernard classifies counseling within three broad categories: intervention, conceptualization, and personalization skills. Intervention skills include strategies, techniques, and actions that counselors use when providing genetic counseling services. Conceptualization skills involve deliberate, strategic thinking and analysis about genetic counseling cases. Personalization skills include subjective reactions during genetic counseling sessions and supervision interactions. Box 10.1 contains examples of psychosocial skills that reflect each category.

Basic helping skills comprise another useful way to think about psychosocial skills. Basic helping skills are essential "tools" in genetic counseling. They "form the foundation of effective genetic counseling relationships . . . and are integral to all aspects of genetic counseling sessions" (McCarthy Veach et al., 2018, p. v). Table 10.1 contains definitions of these skills, and Table 10.2 contains examples of psychosocial responses for each basic skill.

BOX 10.1 Examples of Psychosocial Skills Aligning with the Discrimination Model

Psychosocial Intervention Skills

- Student explains the purpose of genetic counseling in a way the client can understand.
- Student communicates sincerity and genuineness to the client.
- Student moderates their vocal tone and speed to accommodate client emotional state.

Psychosocial Conceptualization Skills

- Student recognizes client physical cues suggesting how the client is feeling.
- Student interprets client verbal and nonverbal cues in deciding to adjust the session plan.
- Student senses additional feelings underlying the client's surface feelings.

Psychosocial Personalization Skills

- Student is able to anticipate their own feelings in new counseling situations.
- Student recognizes genetic counseling situations that may trigger countertransference.
- Student shares their thoughts and feelings about supervisor feedback.

Shugar (2017) proposes a model for teaching genetic counseling students to conceptualize and address patients' psychosocial adaptation. She defines psychosocial adaptation as "the process of coming to terms with the implications of a genetic diagnosis or risk" (p. 218). Viewing a patient's level of psychosocial adaptation on a continuum, Shugar describes four strategies

TABLE 10.1 Genetic Counseling Basic Helping Skill Definitions

Skill	Definition
Physical attending	Counselor uses their body language to communicate understanding and concern for the client.
Psychological attending	Counselor senses experiences through the client's eyes by observing their verbal and nonverbal behaviors and responding to them.
Primary empathy (content)	Counselor reflects surface content of the client's experience.
Primary empathy (affect)	Counselor reflects the client's surface feelings.
Advanced empathy	Counselor communicates their understanding of underlying aspects of the client's experience.
Open-ended question	Counselor requests information the client cannot easily provide with "Yes," "No," or one or two words.
Close-ended question	Counselor requests information the client can easily provide with "Yes," "No," or one or two words.
Confrontation	Counselor challenges client perceptions, beliefs, or viewpoints through a type of feedback that is discrepant from or contrary to the client's self-understanding.
Influence	Counselor expresses their opinion about some aspect of the client's situation.
Advice	Counselor offers suggestions or recommendations about something the client should or should not do.
Information	Counselor provides facts and/or resources relevant to the client's situation.
Self-disclosure	Counselor shares information about themselves.
Self-involving	Counselor expresses their here-and-now feelings about and/or reactions to the client.

Adapted from McCarthy Veach, P., LeRoy, B. S., & Callanan, N. P. (2018). *Facilitating the genetic counseling process: Practice-based skills* (2nd ed.). Springer.

TABLE 10.2 Examples of Basic Helping Skill Responses for a Genetic Counseling Scenario

Client: My husband and my parents have completely different ideas about whether I should have this prenatal test. They keep hounding me about what they think I should do

Skill	Genetic Counselor Response
Physical attending	Counselor maintains eye contact as client speaks.
Psychological attending	"I noticed you are tearing up as you say that."
Primary empathy (content)	"It sounds like you're caught in the middle."
Primary empathy (affect)	"It's upsetting to keep hearing 'do this,' 'do that.'"
Advanced empathy	"It seems like no one has asked you how *you* feel about it?"
Open-ended question	"What do each of them want you to do?"
Close-ended question	"Do you agree more with one of them?"
Confrontation	"And yet you seem to have some ideas about what you want to do."
Influence	"That's a difficult situation to be in."
Advice	"Have you tried asking them for some space to decide?"
Information	"You have about X number of days to decide."
Self-disclosure	"If I were in your situation, I'd be upset, too."
Self-involving	"I'm concerned you might think I'm hounding you, too. I want to be sure we talk about this in a way that you can consider your own thoughts and feelings."

and associated techniques to promote psychosocial adaptation (p. 220):

- *Assess patient adaptation* through contracting, active listening, looking for themes, asking clarifying question, and open physical attending skills.
- *Hypothesize a desired outcome* for the patient through advanced empathy responses; sharing of hypotheses; and assessing informational, emotional, and situational barriers to adaptation.
- *Establish appropriate goals* through primary empathy, reframing, advanced empathy, and immediacy.
- *Reassess patient adaptation* through physical attending skills, checking in with a patient, working collaboratively on a plan, and recognizing the need for follow-up and/or referral.

Shugar (2017, p. 216) recommends students ask themselves four questions:

1. Which issue is my patient most struggling with—adaptation to the risk, to the diagnosis, or to making an informed choice?
2. Where would I intuitively place my patient on a Genetic Counseling Adaptation Continuum (maladapted state ↔ well-adapted state) at this moment in time based on what I have learned from their verbal and nonverbal disclosures?
3. What changes do I hope to see in my patient in the course of today's encounter; what would a better-adapted state look like?
4. What techniques and tools do I have in my toolbox to best help my patient move toward a better-adapted state?

Although patients may be struggling with more than one of these adaptation issues, Shugar recommends students focus on one area when initially building their psychosocial skills.

The ways in which genetic counselors use psychosocial skills will vary across clients and genetic counseling situations, but every situation will involve psychosocial skills of some sort. Djurdjinovic (2009) notes,

> Regardless of how often we are able to engage with a counselee, each connection forms the foundation for a psychological dynamic. The degree to which a [genetic] counselor and patient choose to explore the psychological content within the session will depend on the goals that were mutually set and the skills of the counselor. (p. 167)

Strategies for Building Students' Psychosocial Skills

Fostering students' psychosocial skills is a developmental process that starts at the outset of supervision and continues to the end of the supervision relationship. Several strategies assist in this process.

Discuss Definitions and Perspectives

Building a student's psychosocial skills begins with an initial conversation (which I suggest having early in the supervision relationship). You can start by asking your student what they think psychosocial skills are and why genetic counselors use them. If your student has difficulty expressing their viewpoint, ask them how they would describe genetic counseling to someone who has never heard of it. For a student with previous fieldwork experience, ask how they have seen psychosocial skills used in sessions they observed or in which they participated. Also ask your student what aspects of genetic counseling they like the most and find the most interesting. Their answers to these questions may provide clues about their viewpoint. For example, if their answers emphasize genetic counseling as education, they may be less psychosocially focused.

After your student expresses their perspective, share your thoughts about psychosocial skills and their role in genetic counseling. If your perspectives differ, and they often do, tell students which skills you expect them to demonstrate during the rotation. Encouraging a student to "try things your way" is perfectly appropriate and will be more effective if you provide a context. In other words, as noted by Borders et al. (2006),

> Remind the student that this is . . . [your] own or preferred style of conducting a genetic counseling session, including the use of psychosocial skills, and likely not all aspects of . . . [your] approach will be a match for the student's own personality, cultural makeup, and style. (p. 216)

With regard to stylistic differences, I sometimes use an analogy, telling students that supervision can be like taking a friend with you to purchase clothing. Your friend encourages you to try on items you would never have selected yourself. You try them on, and you discover that some items look good, whereas others do not quite fit.

Students who have completed prior rotation(s) may be inclined to approach psychosocial skills in accordance with the expectations of their former supervisor(s). If your approach differs, refrain from criticizing other supervisors. Instead, frame the differences as stylistic.

Recognize and Address Barriers to Using Psychosocial Skills

As Borders et al. (2006) note, "Genetic counseling students have limited experience applying psychosocial skills, and often are focused on accurate information giving rather than [a] client's nonverbal and verbal cues" (p. 212). Students may also have misperceptions that hinder their development of psychosocial skills. One of your responsibilities as a supervisor is to recognize and address their misperceptions. Common misperceptions and possible supervisor responses include the following:

> *Misperception*: Psychosocial skills are "optional skills," to be used if there is time left at the end of the session.
>
> *Supervisor response*: "To see genetic counseling as linear steps in a process inaccurately deconstructs an interactive dynamic where the psychological is parallel to the genetic and medical discussions" (Djurdjinovic, 2009, p. 167). Work with students to recognize how counselors use psychosocial skills at every point in genetic counseling sessions.
>
> *Misperception*: Psychosocial skills are not as important, interesting, or relevant as genetic information.
>
> *Supervisor response:* Psychosocial skills allow for "the unfolding of genetic and medical information in a psychologically attentive way" (Djurdjinovic, 2009, p. 167). Remind students that skills such as attending and empathy form the basis of all human interactions (McCarthy Veach et al., 2018). Expressing your perspective that the skills are interesting and relevant will help students appreciate their importance.
>
> *Misperception*: Psychosocial skills are too much like psychotherapy and therefore not part of a genetic counselor's role.
>
> *Supervisor response*: Although the skills may be similar to those in psychotherapy, the goals differ. Genetic counselors use these skills to understand and address psychological and social factors that both help and hinder client decision-making and adaptation to their situations (McCarthy Veach et al., 2018).
>
> *Misperception*: Psychosocial skills invade a client's privacy (Borders et al., 2006).

Supervisor response: Inform students that deliberate use of psychosocial skills tailored to a client's situation will help accomplish genetic counseling goals and will not invade their privacy. Point out, for example, that psychosocial responses such as primary and advanced empathy and confrontation, when stated tentatively, preserve a client's right to decline to elaborate and/ or to refute the counselor's statements. Borders et al. (2006) note that

reluctance to address emotional and relational issues may emanate—knowingly or unknowingly—from . . . [a student's] own [life]. . . . These experiences can lead to over-identification with clients and exaggerated emotional responses or opposite responses, such as blind spots, cutting off one's emotions and creating distance between oneself and the client. (p. 212)

Help students reflect on whether the client's discomfort or their own discomfort is influencing their perception and use of psychosocial skills.

Misperception: Psychosocial skills are riskier than genetic information because they are not as straightforward.

Supervisor response: Students may be afraid of opening up client feelings they will not understand or be able to manage, fear their own personal reactions, and/ or think they have to "fix" a client's feelings (Borders et al., 2006; McCarthy Veach et al., 2018). Normalize their fears about managing affect (Borders et al., 2006). Encourage them to talk through their best hopes and worst fears about an upcoming session to help them realistically anticipate what may happen. Discuss and practice strategies for addressing client emotionality. Clarify that the role of a genetic counselor is not to make a client feel better but, rather, to be supportive. Reassure students that you will step in during sessions should it be necessary.

Misperception: A few standard psychosocial responses are sufficient. For example, when a client says they feel it is their fault, the genetic counselor's first (and sometimes only) response should be, "There's nothing you could have done to cause this"; when a client discloses a loss, the counselor should say "I'm sorry" and then shift the topic to something else; and the counselor should complement every client (e.g., praise their parenting skills) even if they do not have evidence to support their statement.

Supervisor response: Explain the distinction between *doing* psychosocial and *being* psychosocial: "*Doing psychosocial* implies a rote application of a learned technique. *Being psychosocial* infers the counselor has adopted a mindset that places psychosocial concerns central to their practice" (Shugar, 2017, p. 216). Role play with students to help them avoid being formulaic or gratuitous. Set goals of taking some "in the moment" risks during sessions rather than using "scripted" responses.

Regardless of which misperceptions a student holds, if they are reluctant or uncomfortable, we suggest you do the following: Empathize with/acknowledge their feelings; validate their belief that psychosocial skills are less concrete and therefore more difficult to prepare for and use; discuss the benefits of trying something new with clients; and remind them that you are there to provide support and guidance during case preparations, counseling sessions, and debriefings. For some students who want to make sure they are saying the "right" thing, it can be helpful to point out there may be many "right" things to say in each situation. You might also share your own challenges using psychosocial skills. Misperceptions can be ingrained, and so you may need more than a single conversation to address them. Importantly, supervisors may hold similar misperceptions (Borders et al., 2006). Therefore, reflection and consultation about your views of psychosocial skills and your comfort using them will help you support students in their skill development.

Assess Student Psychosocial Skills

Identify which psychosocial skill(s) your student is struggling with and make those skills a focus of supervision. Determine whether their skill challenges are more interpersonal (how to interact with the client) or intrapersonal skills (self-awareness and tolerating anxiety) (Hill et al., 2019). Try to pinpoint the source of their difficulty. For example, if a student is having difficulty with empathy, is it because they do not understand the client's feelings, do not know how to communicate their understanding to the client, or are uncertain of what to do after communicating that understanding (McCarthy Veach et al., 2018)?

Set Developmentally Appropriate Goals

Goals involving psychosocial skills should be developmentally appropriate, specific, and positively worded (Borders et al., 2006)—for example, "I will make my questions open-ended when asking clients how they feel." You may need to take a more directive role with novice students in setting goals related to psychosocial skills, helping them identify different types of skills and specific behaviors associated with those skills. In my experience, most students are usually able to demonstrate a higher level of psychosocial skills during case preparation and debriefings than during sessions with clients. Recognizing what to focus on and deciding when and how to respond in actual sessions are challenging for even the most experienced practitioner. Initially, set goals involving less complex skills (e.g., I will communicate my understanding of my patients' feelings about a diagnosis of breast cancer by using primary empathy) and modify them to involve more complex skills as a student progresses (e.g., I will communicate my understanding of my patients' experience of living with a diagnosis of breast cancer by using advanced empathy).

Model Psychosocial Skills

There are two important ways to model psychosocial skills. First, use the way you interact with your student as a model of the psychosocial skills that are relevant for genetic counseling (Wherley et al., 2015). Second, give your student opportunities to observe your counseling sessions. Suggest they pay particular attention to behaviors related to their psychosocial learning goals. For each session they observe, ask your student to briefly note your behaviors, the client's behaviors that seemed to elicit your responses, and the impact of your behaviors on the client. After each session, discuss the student's observations, and share your thoughts and feelings about what transpired in the counseling session. End by asking the student how their observations may affect their own subsequent practice. Note that this strategy might be uncomfortable for you as a supervisor, especially if you are a new supervisor or if a session does not go well. Your willingness to discuss difficult sessions models good self-reflective practice.

Use Directed Self-Reflection Protocols

As described in Chapter 9, directed self-reflection protocols are effective for increasing empathic awareness and for helping students anticipate their feelings, thoughts, and behaviors in challenging clinical situations (Moffett, 2009). Creating a protocol focused on psychosocial skills and psychosocial issues relevant to your site will help build your student's skills.

Assign Psychosocial Case Preparations

Instruct your student to write one or more case preps focused on their speculations about client psychosocial issues and counselor psychosocial issues and interventions. Categories might include the following (McCarthy Veach et al., 2018):

Client Issues

- Motivations for attending genetic counseling or seeking genetic testing
- Feelings about seeing a genetic counselor
- Surface feelings about their situation
- Underlying feelings about their situation
- Thoughts about their situation
- Positive coping strategies
- Negative coping strategies

Counselor (Student) Issues and Interventions

- Feelings the client and their situation may evoke in you
- Psychosocial strategies you may use to manage your feelings
- Client psychosocial issues you may wish to prioritize in order to achieve session goals
- Psychosocial strategies (both interpersonal and intrapersonal) you may use to achieve session goals

Following each counseling session, ask the student to revisit their case prep to modify and/or elaborate it based on what occurred. If a student has difficulty with this assignment, you could independently write a psychosocial case prep and your student could compare it to theirs.

Engage in Role Playing

Role playing is a highly effective strategy for practicing psychosocial skills (McCarthy Veach et al., 2018). When conducted and discussed prior to an actual genetic counseling session, a role play provides anticipatory guidance. When conducted and discussed after a session, a role play offers students an opportunity for a "do over."

If your student is confused about a particular psychosocial skill and/or how to use it, you could play the counselor, thus modeling the skills, and they would play the client. If your student has a reasonable grasp of the skill but feels unsure of themself, have them play the counselor. Role plays can involve actual cases and/or hypothetical ones. For hypothetical cases, you might ask your student to identify a client or situation they find challenging. Recording role plays will facilitate in-depth discussion and allow the student to reflect on them at a later time.

Debrief with Interpersonal Process Recall Methods

As described in Chapter 9, interpersonal process recall (IPR) is a method to help students systematically reflect about counseling interactions with their supervisor (Kagan, 1971; Kagan & Schauble, 1969; Miller et al., 1975). The following questions are useful for eliciting reflections about psychosocial intervention, conceptualization, and personalization skills:

- What did you do? (intervention skills)
- What data from the client (verbal? nonverbal?) was your reaction based on? (intervention skill of psychological attending)
- What were you thinking? (conceptualization and personalization skills)
- What were you feeling? What physical sensations in yourself were you aware of? (personalization skills)
- When else in your interactions with clients have you felt that way? (personalization and conceptualization skills)
- What did you do in those situations? (intervention skills)
- What impact did your actions seem to have on the client? (conceptualization skills)

Focus discussion on the most pivotal portions of a counseling session. Furthermore, to minimize student explanations and justification of their actions, focus them on their thoughts and feelings: "What were you aware of about this client at that moment? What do you think the client wanted from you just then?" (Borders et al., 2006, p. 219). End an IPR discussion about psychosocial skills by having your student respond to the following self-assessment questions (modified from Bannink 2006, pp. 194–195):

- Suppose I was to conduct this session again. What would I do differently or better next time?
- What would the client say I should do differently or better?
- What difference would that have made for the client?
- What difference would that make for me?
- In future sessions when I have clients with similar issues, which psychosocial interventions would I use again? Which wouldn't I?

Use Mind Mapping Methods

To help a student develop a specific psychosocial skill, use a mind map, as described in Chapter 6. Collaborate with the student to identify individual steps (actions, resources, and experiences) they can take to build the skill. The steps will assist with "successive approximation"—that is, each step comprises an opportunity for success to build student confidence and move the student toward mastery of the skill. Figure 10.1 illustrates an example of a mind map for empathic understanding, which is one component of empathy.

Connect Psychosocial Skills to Their Effects

Feedback Strategies

When giving your student feedback about their psychosocial skills, link their behavior to its effects on session processes and/ or outcomes. This approach will help them more fully understand the significance of psychosocial skills in genetic counseling. You can begin by asking the student their perceptions of the effects

Goal: Increase student empathic understanding

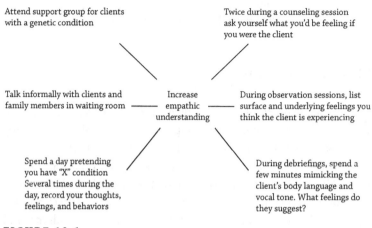

FIGURE 10.1

Mind mapping example.

(evocative approach; see Chapter 7). Then, share your impressions (e.g., "When you stayed silent for a while when the patient was crying, it gave them space to experience their sadness").

Consider using a rating form for psychosocial skills during counseling sessions for later debriefing discussions. You can either create your own form or use one of several counseling skills rating forms available on the internet (e.g., fillable online Heidelberg Basic Counseling Skills Rating Sheet [https://www.pdffiller.com]).

Journaling

Encourage your student to maintain a weekly journal in which they respond to these questions with particular attention to their psychosocial skills (Bannink, 2006, p. 199):

- What was my best session recently?
- What made it such a good session?

- How did I do that?
- What does that say about me?
- How will I be able to do that more often (or again)?

Closing Thoughts

As with all aspects of student development, a thoughtful, non-judgmental, and collaborative approach is critical for fostering psychosocial skills. Carefully consider what to realistically expect from students based on their current developmental level (Borders et al., 2006), and encourage them to do the same. A participant in a study of master genetic counselors (Miranda et al., 2016) expressed a perspective that I believe is applicable for both students and supervisors: "My job is to do the best job I can, not necessarily to think about what was the best I've ever done . . . sometimes it does go badly, and you just deal with that. . . . Nobody is perfect. Nobody is going to fix everything" (p. 775).

Learning Activities

Most learning activities can be adapted for dyad or small group discussions or for written exercises. Time estimates are provided for discussions, but additional time should be allotted for large group processing.

Activity 10.1 Addressing Student Misperceptions About Psychosocial Skills

Individually write a response to address each of these student misperceptions. Write as if you are speaking directly to the student.

Student: I think of psychosocial skills as "optional skills," to be used if there is time left at the end of the session.

Your response:

Student: I don't think psychosocial skills are as important or relevant as genetic information.

Your response:

Student: I'm not supposed to be doing psychotherapy.

Your response:

Student: I don't want to invade a client's privacy.

Your response:

Student: Psychosocial skills are too risky because they're not as straightforward as genetic information.

Your response:

Student: Aren't a few standard psychosocial responses sufficient?

Your response:

Student: It feels like we are just chatting!

Your response:

Share your individual responses with a partner or in small groups.

Estimated time: 35 minutes

Activity 10.2 Psychosocial Case Preparations

In small specialty groups or with a partner:

Part I: Write three to five brief role-play scenarios involving common client psychosocial issues at your site.

Estimated time: 20 minutes

Part II: Using one of the scenarios you developed, create a psychosocial case prep to serve as a model for students. You can refer to categories of client psychosocial issues and counselor psychosocial issues and interventions listed in this chapter to develop the case prep.

Estimated time: 20 minutes

Activity 10.3 Directed Self-Reflection Protocol

In small specialty groups, generate 15 questions you could ask a student to reflect upon regarding psychosocial skills that are relevant to your practice specialty. Try to include questions about *intervention* skills (e.g., How would you respond to a mother who bursts into tears upon learning her child's testing confirms the diagnosis of fragile X syndrome?), *conceptualization* skills (e.g., When counseling a prenatal couple, what do you think might prompt a father to say he'd go along with whatever the mother decides about testing? How do you think the mother might feel about his answer?), and *personalization* skills (How would you feel talking to a 25-year-old man about his risk for colon cancer?).

Estimated time: 20 minutes

Adapted from Moffett, L. (2009). Directed self-reflection protocols in supervision. *Training and Education in Professional Psychology, 3,* 78–83.

Activity 10.4 Mind Mapping

With a partner or in small groups, identify a specific psychosocial skill and then create a mind map to help a student develop the skill [*Hint*: see Figure 10.1 for an example]:

- Write the skill in the center of your paper.
- Draw spokes around the skill.
- List one step at the end of each spoke for helping a student build the skill.

Estimated time: 25 minutes

Note: This activity can be expanded to create three mind maps— one for an intervention skill, one for a conceptualization skill, and one for a personalization skill.

Activity 10.5 Addressing Students' Use of Psychosocial Skills: Triad Role Plays

Triads take turns as supervisor, student, and observer for the following scenarios. After each role play, the observer and student give feedback to the supervisor about how they addressed the issue with the student. [*Hint*: Supervisors may wish to use IPR questions, if appropriate, to focus their discussion with the student.]

Scenario: The supervisor and student are debriefing a session in which the client learned they carry the gene for retinitis pigmentosa. Upon learning the test result, the client said, "Why did this happen?" At that point, the student explained the genetic cause of the condition. The supervisor thinks the student missed the client's actual concern of "Why did this happen *to me*?" and now wants to address this with the student.

Adapted from Djurdjinovic, L. (2009). Psychosocial counseling. In W. R. Uhlmann, J. L. Schuette, & B. Yashar (Eds.), *A guide to genetic counseling* (2nd ed., pp. 133–176). Wiley.

Scenario: The supervisor and student are debriefing a prenatal session for a client whose prenatal testing results were positive for trisomy 13. During the session, the client began to cry and said, "Oh, my poor baby. I was really hoping everything would turn out to be okay. I can't stand that this is happening to her. I don't know how I'll get through this." The student responded by saying, "We are stronger than we think." The supervisor wants to discuss the student's response.

Adapted from Keppers, R., McCarthy Veach, P., MacFarlane, I. M., Schema, L., & LeRoy, B. S. (2022). Differences in genetic counseling student responses to intense patient affect: A study of genetic counseling graduate students training in North American programs. *Journal of Genetic Counseling, 31*(2), 398–410. https://doi.org/10.1002/jgc4.1505.

Scenario: The student and supervisor are debriefing a prenatal session for a client whose non-invasive prenatal test and level 2 ultrasound findings were consistent with trisomy 18. The student was discussing with the client whether she wished to pursue amniocentesis when the client said, "I don't know. [Pause] God makes everything possible. Only God knows what can happen. We leave things in his hands." The student then said, "Do you feel that you wish to discuss this with someone in your religious community?" The supervisor wants to discuss the student's response.

Adapted from Sitaula, A., McCarthy Veach, P., MacFarlane, I.M., Lee, W., & Redlinger-Grosse, K. (2022). Genetic counselors' response types to prenatal patient deferring or attributing religious/spiritual statements: An exploratory study of US genetic counselors. *Journal of Genetic Counseling*. doi.org/10.1002/jgc4.1634

Estimated time: 45 minutes

Note: If you process this exercise with the larger group, include discussion about the extent to which the supervisor in each scenario focused on the student's intervention skills, conceptualization skills, and/or personalization skills.

11

Ethics and Professionalism in Supervision

PATRICIA MCCARTHY VEACH

Objectives

- Describe supervisor responsibilities regarding ethical and professional supervision.
- Identify common ethical and professional issues in genetic counseling supervision.
- Suggest strategies to promote ethical and professional practice in the supervisory relationship.

Supervisor Responsibilities

The National Society of Genetic Counselors' (NSGC, 2018) Code of Ethics states that "genetic counselors' professional relationships with other genetic counselors, trainees, employees, employers and other professionals are based on mutual respect, caring, collaboration, fidelity, veracity and support" (p. 7). Activities contributing to ethical and professional supervision relationships with students include the following:

- Sharing knowledge and providing mentorship and guidance for students' professional development
- Respecting and valuing students' knowledge, perspectives, contributions, and areas of competence
- Encouraging student ethical behavior
- Ensuring students undertake responsibilities commensurate with their knowledge, experience, and training
- Maintaining appropriate boundaries to avoid exploitation of students

Ethical supervision is a major competency domain for genetic counseling supervisors (Eubanks Higgins et al., 2013; see also Chapter 1, Appendix 1A). Box 11.1 lists specific competencies describing supervisor ethical conduct.

Ethical Considerations in Clinical Supervision

Barnett and Molzon (2014) identify several ethical issues in clinical supervision, including informed consent (which in genetic counseling takes the form of a supervision agreement), modeling, multiple relationships, and boundary crossings and violations.

Supervision Agreement

In psychology, a supervision relationship involves an informed consent process. In genetic counseling, a supervision agreement is often informal but an essential part of the process (see Chapter 3). According to Barnett and Molzon (2014), supervision agreement topics should include

---

This chapter focuses on ethics and professionalism in the supervisory relationship and not in genetic counseling practice. There are multiple resources on the latter topic.

BOX 11.1 Genetic Counselor Supervisor Ethical Supervision Competencies

Professional Conduct

Genetic counselor supervisors:
- Are ethical in practice and supervision
- Demonstrate ethical and professional standards of genetic counseling practice (e.g., confidentiality, duty to warn)
- Seek appropriate consultation in situations of ethical uncertainty
- Demonstrate knowledge of the professional Code of Ethics of relevant professional organizations such as the National Society of Genetic Counselors (NSGC) and Canadian Association of Genetic Counsellors (CAGC)
- Communicate an understanding of legal and regulatory documents and their impact on the profession (e.g., HIPPA, informed consent)

Nature and Boundaries of Supervision

Genetic counselor supervisors:
- Communicate knowledge of ethical considerations that pertain to the supervisory relationship (e.g., multiple role relationships, due process, confidentiality)
- Clearly define the boundaries of the supervisory relationship
- Avoid simultaneous roles in addition to supervision with students (i.e., teacher, research mentor, employer, friend) or monitor them for negative effects on students when unavoidable
- Maintain confidentiality from those outside the site about student evaluation and feedback
- Explain the rationale and/or boundaries around addressing the student's personal issues during the supervision process

Source: Eubanks Higgins, S., McCarthy Veach, P., MacFarlane, I. M., Borders, L. D., LeRoy, B. S., & Callanan, N. (2013) Genetic counseling supervisor competencies: Results of a Delphi study. *Journal of Genetic Counseling, 22*, 39–57 (p. 56). Reprinted with permission from the *Journal of Genetic Counseling.*

expectations, responsibilities, and obligations of both super-visor and supervisee . . . scheduling and emergency contact information; documentation [requirements]; . . . evaluation and feedback . . . [and] expectations and requirements for successful completion of the training experience; expec-tations for confidentiality and . . . reasonably anticipated limits to confidentiality; legal requirements . . .; [and] expec-tations for use of the supervisor and when the supervisee should contact [them]. (pp. 1052–1053)

Including these elements means the supervision agreement sets not just expectations around logistics but also expectations around professional and ethical behaviors for both the supervisor and student.

Modeling

"More is caught than taught" . . .our supervisees watch us very closely. Whether we like it or not, whether we are aware of it or not, our supervisees learn more about practice from the way we work with them than from what we say about their actual practice.
—SHULMAN (2006, P. 24)

Supervisors are role models for ethical and legal responsi-bility (American Psychological Association, 2014): "One of the supervisor's tasks is to provide professional socialization, to not only cultivate skills but also instill professional conscience. Certainly, modeling professional behavior is one way of teaching it" (Dewane, 2007, p. 35). The ways supervisors interact with students, clients, and others may be more influential than what they say (Barnett & Molzon, 2014). Barnett and Molzon (2014) provide examples of a supervisor who stresses the importance of confidentiality but discusses sensitive information about clients and students in a busy hallway. They assert that these behaviors will affect students' views of who counselors and supervisors are and what they do. They further note that supervisor behaviors in supervision sessions are impactful: "If the supervisor is warm, empathic, and understanding (or cold, emotionally distant, and unsupportive, for that matter) . . . [students] may internalize these qualities and emulate them in relationships with clients, both now and in the future, as well as with their future supervisees" (p. 1055). Borders et al. (2006) note that "ultimately, supervisors should be aware that they are modeling at every moment the student is at the site. Supervisors are constantly modeling professional behavior, including how they talk about clients, the medical staff, and genetic counseling colleagues" (p. 217).

Multiple Relationships

Supervisors are not only responsible for increasing student awareness of boundary issues with clients but also role models regarding management of boundaries in supervision (Barnett & Molzon, 2014; Gu et al., 2011). A common boundary issue involves multiple relationships. Multiple relationships refer to instances in which a supervisor has a primary professional role with a student and at least one other, significantly different role with them. These roles can be concurrent or consecutive (Gu et al., 2011). Genetic counselor supervisors often have more than one academic/professional relationship with a student (e.g., member of the student's graduate committee or course instructor), and these are generally viewed as appropriate. Multiple relationships also refer to intimate, social, and/or therapeutic relationships that supervisors may have with a student. Intimate, social, and therapeutic relationships should be avoided at least for the duration of the supervision relationship because they pose a direct boundary violation and place the student in a vulnerable position.

Multiple professional relationships generally are less problematic than other types of relationships, but they are not without ethical risk. Two major criteria determine whether a multiple relationship of any sort is unethical: the likelihood it will impair the supervisor's judgment and the risk that it will lead to exploitation of the student. Either of these criteria is sufficient for raising questions of ethical appropriateness.

Boundary Crossings and Boundary Violations

Because different relationships "have different goals and tasks, they may lead to numerous boundary crossings and boundary violations" (Gu et al., 2011, p. 36). *Boundary crossings* are behaviors that are "departures from the strictest professional role and they may or may not benefit supervisees" (p. 35). An example of a boundary crossing is taking a student to a professional meeting. *Boundary violations* are behaviors "outside the limits of commonly accepted practice and may place supervisees at significant risk" (p. 35). An example of a boundary violation is asking a student to babysit one's children.

Risks Posed by Boundary Crossings and Violations

Gu and colleagues (2011) investigated genetic counseling supervisors', non-supervisors', and students' awareness of ethical behaviors related to establishing and maintaining clear supervisor–student boundaries. Participants reported academic/professional and social boundary crossings and violations that posed one or more risks:

> *Risk of exploitation.* Given the evaluative nature of supervision, students are unavoidably in a less powerful position and therefore at greater risk of feeling coerced to comply.
> For example, "My supervisor asked me to house sit and care for pets multiple times while I was a student. I had a harder time saying 'No' when I knew [they were] my supervisor and would be evaluating my counseling skills" (Genetic counselor; Gu et al., 2011, unpublished data).

Time of vulnerability. Students are in the process of developing a professional identity and may be more "susceptible" to incorporating a supervisor's ethically questionable practices.

Loss of objectivity. When a supervisor and student have a social relationship, they may lose their ability to evaluate the supervision experience, and the supervisor may lose their ability to evaluate the student's genetic counseling skills in an unbiased manner. Neither party may want to discuss issues that will hurt their social relationship.

> For example, "One of my colleagues (a new grad we hired) had a personal friendship with one of the students (established when they were both students). That colleague was consistently giving the student an overly favorable evaluation compared to everyone else's assessment of her performance, and we were concerned that it was because of the friendship" (Genetic counselor; Gu et al., 2011, unpublished data).

Creates rivalry. Peers may believe the student is receiving special treatment.

Provides poor modeling. The supervisor's behaviors set an undesirable example for students and for colleagues.

Causes role conflicts. The student may become confused about the boundaries around supervision (e.g., Are you my supervisor or my friend?).

> For example, "[When they were a student, their supervisor was undergoing a major life event] . . . I was trying to be a good friend because she seemed to have no one else to support her. I didn't know how to draw boundaries when my own supervisor was reaching out for advice from me. . . . I got a really high evaluation for that clinical rotation, and until this day I'm not really sure if it was deserved, or if it was a 'thank you' gesture" (Genetic counselor; Gu et al., 2011, p. 44).

Reduces supervisor credibility. Students and colleagues may perceive the supervisor as less expert and trustworthy.

Additional Issues

Some research has identified supervisor behaviors that lack professionalism and may constitute a failure to uphold ethical standards of supervision practice. Watkins (1997) described "ineffective" supervisors as "intolerant, nonempathic, discouraging, defensive, and uninterested in training or consultation to improve their supervisory skills" (as cited in Magnuson et al., 2000, p. 189). Magnuson and colleagues (2000) interviewed practicing counselors about poor supervisor behaviors they encountered as supervisees. Magnuson et al. identified experiences consistent with six "overarching principles":

> *Imbalance*: Supervisor gives uneven attention to various aspects of supervision.
>
> *Developmentally inappropriate*: Supervisor is not sensitive and responsive to students' changing developmental needs.
>
> *Intolerance of differences*: Supervisor lacks flexibility in their supervision approach.
>
> *Poor model of professionalism*: Supervisor does not provide sufficient support and guidance and/or behaves unethically.
>
> *Untrained*: Supervisor is not prepared to address difficult supervision situations effectively.
>
> *Professionally apathetic*: Supervisor lacks commitment to working with students.

Magnuson et al. further classified supervisor behaviors within three spheres (p. 195):

> *Organizational–administrative* (e.g., fails to clarify expectations, provide standards for accountability, assess supervisee needs, and/or be adequately prepared for supervision interactions)
>
> *Technical–cognitive* (e.g., engages in behaviors suggestive of an unskilled practitioner, supervisor, and/or unreliable

resource professional; provides vague feedback; does not appreciate student's perspective)

Relational–affective (e.g., does not provide a safe supervision environment; gives too much or too little corrective or positive feedback; is insensitive to the student's learning needs; avoids issues between the student and themself)

Strategies to Promote Ethical and Professional Supervision Practice

This section describes strategies to promote supervisor professional and ethical supervision practices to maximize the effectiveness of supervision and minimize unintended negative consequences for students.

Make a Lifelong Commitment to Ethical Awareness, Sensitivity, and Behavior

All professionals, supervisors or not, have the capacity to succumb to ethical weaknesses and misjudgments . . .the importance of establishing and maintaining strong professional ethics throughout one's career should not be discounted.

—CIMINO ET AL. (2013, P. 55)

Three types of professional development activities contribute to ethical practice.

Self-Reflection

Engage in self-reflection when ethical situations arise. Examine your feelings, thoughts, and behaviors in these situations. The more you use self-reflection to know yourself, the greater the likelihood you will practice ethically. As a master genetic

282 | CLINICAL SUPERVISION IN GENETIC COUNSELING

counselor noted (Miranda et al., 2016), a critical element of practice is

> having a superior [self] understanding . . . a much more in-depth sort of therapeutic understanding of who we are, how we were raised, what our biases and values and beliefs are, and how that imposes [on] and informs our work and [how they] can be barriers. (p. 772)

Consultation and Supervision

Best supervisor practices include ongoing peer supervision/consultation (Borders, 2014). Participation in regular peer supervision and consultation serves as a dependable resource for discussing ethical issues. This can include one-to-one mentoring related to supervision or peer supervision groups focused on supervision skills (see Chapter 15).

Continuing Education

Take advantage of continuing education opportunities (Borders, 2014). They will enhance your reflection about ethical and professional practice.

Set and Maintain Clear Boundaries Around the Supervision Relationship

I have often felt very uncomfortable in terms of not knowing where the boundaries should be in the supervisor–supervisee relationship, especially as different supervisors have different feelings regarding what that relationship should be . . . I definitely do recall [as a student] being constantly on edge, unsure if my own actions were appropriate.

—GENETIC COUNSELOR (GU ET AL., 2011, P. 43)

Clarify boundaries. Discuss boundaries with your student as part of initiating the supervision relationship and throughout supervision, as necessary. It is the supervisor's responsibility to clearly outline and maintain these boundaries because the student is in a vulnerable position.

Maintain a Distinction Between a Friendly Relationship and a Friendship

Usually forming a friendly relationship (in clinic-only) with a student is sometimes hard "not" to do, but then I just do not do anything socially with the student until the supervision is over. I think I have always waited until after graduation.
— GENETIC COUNSELOR (GU ET AL., 2011, UNPUBLISHED DATA)

Genetic counselors who regularly supervise students should consider limiting social interactions with students throughout their training because it may be unclear which students they will supervise. Related to this distinction, I suggest you carefully consider the potential risks of friending students on social media sites. As a genetic counselor (Gu et al., 2011, unpublished data) noted,

As a soon to be supervisor I am more aware of online networking websites. . . .I was "friends" with some of my supervisors on these networks which allowed the supervisor access to a lot of personal information and pictures (marital status, sexual orientation, religious views, political views, etc.). In turn, I had access to a lot of the supervisors' personal information. I believe that use of these websites blurs the boundary between being "friendly" with students and being professional."

Respect and Protect Student Rights Regarding Confidentiality and Privacy

I felt that my supervisor would often share personal details about my cases and supervision with my classmates without explicit permission. This was based on the fact that my supervisor shared such details about my classmates with me or in classes I attended. In order to resolve the situation, I was very guarded about the things I said in supervision, always making sure that they were things I would not mind being shared with others.

—GENETIC COUNSELOR (GU ET AL., 2011, P. 43)

Including a section on confidentiality and its limits in a supervision agreement will emphasize your intent to act with discretion where student and client information are concerned and help you avoid situations such as the following: "My classmates and I had several situations where supervisors would . . . ask personal questions not pertaining to their supervisory role. . . . We did our best to avoid discussing personal information about ourselves and each other" (Genetic counselor; Gu et al., 2011, unpublished data).

Limit your requests for student personal information to a "need to know" basis—that is, to information relevant to their performance and professional development. Explain why you are requesting personal information because students may misunderstand the reason. Be mindful of the amount of time you spend in casual conversation with a student because extensive conversations may breach their right to privacy.

There may be times when personal factors are relevant to a case or a rotation. For example, a student and supervisor may come from different cultural backgrounds, causing them to interpret a client's comments differently (particularly if the client is similar in cultural background to either the student or the supervisor). In these instances, it is important for the supervisor and student to discuss the origins of their different perspectives. The supervisor should, however, explicitly state that the student may set their own boundaries on what they share or discuss related to personal identity and maintain confidentiality for anything the student shares (see strategies for incorporating cultural identities into supervision discussed in Chapter 4).

Manage Multiple Relationships in an Ethical Manner

Engage mindfully in multiple professional relationships. Consider potential benefits and risks of multiple relationships with students in order to make deliberate decisions about entering into them. Gu et al. (2011, p. 47) suggest supervisors use the following model (Burian & O'Connor-Slimp, 2000):

- Begin by asking yourself
  - Is the additional relationship necessary or should I avoid it?
  - Can it potentially cause harm [professional and/or personal] to the student?
  - If harm seems unlikely or avoidable, would the additional relationship prove beneficial?
  - Is there a risk the multiple relationship could disrupt the supervisory relationship?
  - Can I evaluate the matter objectively?
- Next, reflect on internal clues: "Is the issue eliciting strong feelings in me? Do I feel reluctant to discuss the situation with colleagues? Whose needs are being met?" (Gu et al., 2011, p. 47).
- Then, re-evaluate "possible risks and benefits to the student, [yourself], classmates, other co-workers, and the training program . . . inform the student of the potential harm of a multiple relationship . . . and inform the director of the student's training program" (Gu et al., 2011, p. 47).

Compartmentalize Activities Associated with Each Professional Relationship

Over the years, I have had many supervisees and have taught one of the classes for the Genetic Counseling program. So, for the majority of my supervisees, I have had multiple relationships. I found it critical to separate my "class" evaluations from "clinical," and make the student aware that I would be evaluating them on two separate categories. At times, I have had similar critiques for students in my class as in my clinical evals, but I do not think that it is fair to evaluate performances contra laterally.

  —GENETIC COUNSELOR (GU ET AL., 2011, UNPUBLISHED DATA)

Keep tasks and evaluations for multiple professional relationships as separate as possible. Inform the student of your intention to do so. In addition, be mindful of times when multiple roles may lead you to treat a particular student differently so this can be minimized. For example, a supervisor who is also working on a student's research project may be tempted to limit the number of clients the student sees because the supervisors wants the student to focus their time on research. Recognition of "competing" motivations will help the supervisor avoid decreasing the student's cases. Early identification of potential areas of conflict can help lessen adverse effects of multiple professional relationships.

Avoid Nonprofessional Relationships with Students

I had a situation in which I . . . developed a close personal relationship with this supervisor. . . . [One day] . . . I felt that I could be open with her about some of the struggles I was having in my sessions, and I asked her for some more specific comments on feedback that I had been getting. She told me that I was being "defensive" . . . I felt hurt and confused by her reaction.

  —GENETIC COUNSELING STUDENT

  (GU ET AL., 2011, P. 44)

When possible, avoid forming a nonprofessional relationship, and suspend a pre-existing one, when you are supervising a student.

Cultivate a Personal Support Network

[When I was] a student supervisee, a supervisor who was over-stressed and unhappy in her job spent a lot of time complaining to me.
—GENETIC COUNSELOR (GU ET AL., 2011, P. 43)

Develop a social support network to prevent using students as a "sounding board" for personal situations and to avoid crossing a boundary into friendship while you are supervising. Although it can be instructive to model self-reflection about how you, as a supervisor, handled professional situations, avoid complaining or looking to students for validation.

Delineate and Enforce Your Expectations of Students

One of your supervisory responsibilities involves establishing reasonable expectations about student behavior and holding students to those expectations (Eubanks Higgins et al., 2013; Worthington et al., 2002). Although setting expectations can be relatively easy, they may be challenging to "enforce." The more you value autonomy and self-direction as part of students' developmental processes, the more difficult you may find it to assert your power as a supervisor. Realize, however, that autonomy and self-direction "may be 'trumped' by [the] need to set and maintain clear performance expectations and to place limits on [student] behavior" (McCarthy Veach et al., 2012, p. 221). Monitor your "ambivalence about power," and recognize situations requiring you to exert your influence (McCarthy Veach et al., 2012).

Develop a Strong Supervisory Working Alliance

Build a trusting and open relationship with clearly agreed upon goals and tasks. Address cultural factors (see Chapter 4), and pay attention to student well-being (see Chapter 12). Creating a safe and open environment in which students are able to freely share their thoughts and feelings can maximize their professional development (Barnett & Molzon, 2014). As Worthington et al. (2002) note, a critical aspect of supervision is "facilitation of professional development within a flexible and understanding atmosphere while . . . [also holding students] accountable for the achievement of standards corresponding to their level of training (p. 348).

Closing Thoughts

When you provide supervision in an ethical and professional manner, you are a powerful source of the support and guidance necessary for student growth. What you do and say as a supervisor have considerable influence. Committing to engage in deliberate supervision best practices will serve you well in behaving ethically and professionally. I think the following quote captures the essence of ethical and professional behavior:

The most pressing ethical question is to make sure that everything you do from a scientific standpoint is done for the ultimate good and positive issue for the people that you're caring about.
—DR. ANTHONY FAUCI (BRAINY QUOTES, N.D.-A)

Learning Activities

Most learning activities can be adapted for dyad or small group discussions or for written exercises. Time estimates are provided for discussions, but additional time should be allotted for large group processing.

Activity 11.1 Addressing Student Questions About Ethical and Legal Aspects of Supervision

In small groups, discuss how you would address each of the following questions from students:

- What are the key ethical considerations in the supervision relationship?
- How do supervisors go about setting and managing boundaries in supervision?
- What are examples of appropriate/inappropriate boundaries?
- How do supervisors manage multiple relationships with students (e.g., teacher and supervisor)?
- How appropriate is supervisor–student contact (social) outside of the workplace setting?
- How much should a supervisor encourage self-disclosure by the student? To what degree should personal lives of the supervisor/student be disclosed?
- How do supervisors deal with students' emotions (sadness, anger, etc.) without it turning into a counseling session?

Estimated time: 30 minutes

Activity 11.2 Boundaries in Supervision Discussion

Consider each of the following supervisor behaviors. Select the number that best reflects your opinion about how appropriate each behavior is. There are no right or wrong answers.

Scale: 1 = Never appropriate; 2 = Appropriate under rare conditions; 3 = Appropriate under some conditions; 4 = Appropriate under most conditions; 5 = Always appropriate; NS = Not sure.

- Supervisor invites student to "hang out" (dinner, sightseeing) during a national meeting.
- Supervisor asks the student what they think about their classmates.

- Supervisor takes personal phone calls in their office while discussing cases with a student.
- Supervisor gives the student their cell phone and home phone numbers.
- Supervisor invites the entire office staff, including the student, out for happy hour to overcome a tough day.
- Supervisor invites/expects the student to have lunch with supervisors in the lunchroom.
- Supervisor uses example of another classmate's counseling skills to explain what they expect of the student.
- Supervisor accepts the student's "friend request" on a social media site.
- Supervisor advises a colleague not to hire the student for a research assistantship because the student needs to work on their rotation tasks.
- Supervisor gives the student dating advice.

Next, share your answers in small groups.

Estimated time: 40 minutes

Adapted from Gu, L., McCarthy Veach, P., Eubanks, S., LeRoy, B. S., & Callanan, N. (2011). Boundary issues and multiple relationships in genetic counseling supervision: Supervisor, non-supervisor, and student perspectives. *Journal of Genetic Counseling, 20*, 35–48.

Activity 11.3 Strategies for Addressing Boundary Issues in Supervision

In small groups:

- List the boundary issues you have encountered or think you may encounter in providing supervision.
- For each of these boundary issues, discuss and list strategies for addressing it.
- Specifically, what action(s) would you take?

Estimated time: 30 minutes

Note: Remind participants not to share any information that is identifying.

Activity 11.4 Addressing Ethical Situations: Triad Role Plays

Triads take turns as supervisor, student, and observer for the following scenarios. After each role play, the observer and student give feedback to the supervisor about how they addressed the issue with the student.

Scenarios

- When your student went to the waiting room to bring a client back for the session, they introduced themself, saying, "I will be your genetic counselor today." They never disclosed they are a student. A staff member overhead the exchange and told you about it.
- Your student told you that another of their supervisors in the rotation is extremely harsh in giving feedback. The student says they are feeling very discouraged and hope you can do something about how that supervisor is treating them.
- Your student asks if it would be ok to use part of the supervision meeting to talk about their distress over their impending divorce.
- Your student shows you a follow-up letter they drafted for a client. The client's name and date of service are wrong, and the genetic information is inaccurate in several places. You suspect the student cut and pasted sections of a follow-up letter for a previous client.
- Your student looked at the medical records of one of their family members who received services at your site. You learned about this from another staff member who overheard the student talking about it with a classmate.

- Your student was in the clinic when a genetic counselor from another institution came in for care in follow up to a miscarriage. The student discussed this with the other students in their class and relayed the discussion to you.

Estimated time: 10 minutes per role play; 10 minutes per debriefing each role play

Activity 11.5 Ethical Decision-Making

Use the following questions to work through one of the situations in Learning Activity 11.2. List each question and indicate your response. Then discuss your responses with a partner.

- What is the concern or dilemma?
- Who do you anticipate will be affected by the decision?
- What ethical supervision standard(s) is relevant?
- What personal feelings, biases, or self-interest might affect your decision in this situation?
- Are there social, cultural, religious, or similar factors that are pertinent to the situation?
- What alternative courses of action are there?
- What will you decide to do?

Estimated time: 30 minutes

Note: A different situation can be selected for this exercise.

Adapted from Pope, K. S., & Vasquez, M. J. T. (2010). *Ethics in psychotherapy and counseling: A practical guide*. Wiley.

12

Promoting Student Wellness

PATRICIA MCCARTHY VEACH

Objectives

- Define wellness.
- Identify self-care as a component of wellness.
- Discuss the role of supervision in student wellness.
- Review strategies for promoting wellness and self-care.

What Is Wellness?

To take adequate care of ourselves, we must continue learning throughout life what facilitates, deepens, and strengthens our personal sense of well-being and peace of mind.

—BAKER (2003, P. 59)

Wellness pertains to all aspects of an individual's life and is synergistic, multifaceted, and best characterized as a continuum (Lenz & Smith, 2010). Wellness refers to an orientation toward optimal well-being that involves integration of body, mind, and spirit (Myers et al., 2000). Myers et al. (2000) created a model in which they identify seven wellness domains: emotional, intellectual, physical, social, environmental, financial, and spiritual. Two of the domains in their model are especially relevant to genetic counseling supervision: emotional (recognizing and managing one's feelings) and intellectual (remaining curious and open to learning). Of the many factors contributing to wellness, resilience and self-care are noteworthy and are discussed next.

Resilience

Resilience is the ability of individuals to recover from or adjust easily to aversive events and/or to any type of change (Merriam-Webster, n.d.-a). Wells et al. (2016) interviewed genetic counselors about the meaning they derive from their work. Many counselors identified resilience as critical to their development and experience of meaning in their practice. Miranda et al. (2016) found that master genetic counselors draw upon their personal resilience to cope with the emotional intensity of their work.

Hou and Skovholt (2020) studied highly resilient therapists and found they share common characteristics. These characteristics are reflected in studies of genetic counselors (e.g., Miranda et al., 2016; Wells et al., 2016). Box 12.1 contains a list of common characteristics as described by Hou and Skovholt (2020).

Self-Care

Self-care is giving the world the best of you rather than what's left of you.

—KATIE REED (ANQUOTES, N.D.)

Self-care is essential for improving and maintaining wellness. Self-care is "a set of purposeful behavioral strategies that promote the well-being of the self but also help to reduce stress and overcome challenges that enable the worker to engage effectively with their clients" (Acker, 2018, p. 715). Baker (2003) identifies three self-care components: self-awareness, self-regulation, and balance. She describes *self-awareness* as observing one's "physical and psychological experience to the degree possible without

BOX 12.1 Characteristics of Resilient Therapists

Resilient therapists possess a framework of core values and beliefs involving
- a personal values/beliefs base;
- trust, faith, patience, and acceptance of ambiguity;
- hopefulness, positivity, and optimism; and
- gratitude, appreciation, and honor.

Resilient therapists are drawn to strong interpersonal relationships such that they
- are strongly connected to personal relationships;
- stay connected to valuable professional relationships;
- have compassion for others;
- feel loved and supported;
- are humble, open, and vulnerable to feedback; and
- experience love, kindness, and compassion.

Resilient therapists desire to learn and grow, and as such
- desire ongoing intellectual development;
- are committed to ongoing personal growth;
- possess curiosity;
- are persistent, determined, and dedicated; and
- engage in intentional self-reflection and self-awareness.

Resilient therapists actively engage with self, resulting in
- self-knowledge;
- compassion for self;
- vocational conviction;
- a self-conservation mode;
- self-acceptance and contentment;
- authenticity and valuing equality between people;
- courage;
- generosity expressed in boundaried ways;
- assertiveness in creating a balanced and fulfilling personal life;
- humor; and
- playfulness, lightheartedness, and creativity.

Source: Hou, J. M., & Skovholt, T. M. (2020). Characteristics of highly resilient therapists. *Journal of Counseling Psychology*, 67, 386–400.

distortion or avoidance" (p. 15). She notes that self-awareness takes effort because it requires an individual to recognize their internal struggles to manage differing needs. Baker describes *self-regulation* as "conscious and less conscious management of our physical and emotional impulses, drives, and anxieties" (p. 15). Self-regulation ability increases the more self-aware an individual is of their internal processes and the more they attempt to manage them. Baker characterizes *balance* as involving "many factors such as time, energy, and money. Balance is actually a high-level function involving modulation and oscillation. The process entails searching for the center on the continuum between the extremes" (p. 16).

The Role of Supervision in Promoting Student Wellness and Self-Care

Stress and Distress

There's so much to know, and I can never seem to remember it all, no matter how hard I try. I also always feel like I'll never get caught up with knowledge and it makes me feel inadequate.

—GENETIC COUNSELING STUDENT
(JUNGBLUTH ET AL., 2011, P. 280)

I have felt often that I can't be open and honest with the course coordinators or other tutors or supports, because ultimately one day I might be working for them and I don't want to appear weak or incompetent. . . . I feel like I am being constantly judged, and that gives me a lot of stress.

—GENETIC COUNSELING STUDENT
(JUNGBLUTH ET AL., 2011, P. 280)

Stress and distress pose threats to an individual's wellness and functioning. *Stress* is a state of mental or emotional strain or tension resulting from adverse or demanding circumstances

(Merriam-Webster, n.d.-b). Stress involves "a relationship between the person and the environment that is appraised by the person as relevant to his or her well-being and in which the person's resources are taxed or exceeded" (Folkman & Lazarus, 1985, p. 152). Stress can be acute or chronic, situational or cumulative (Baker, 2003, p. 19). *Distress* is an individual's subjective emotional response to stressors (Barnett & Molzon, 2014). When inadequately managed, distress can lead to diminished clinical performance. Relatedly, when human services professionals fail to make their own needs for health, self-care, balance, and wellness a priority, they jeopardize their ability to manage stress and are at risk for burnout and compassion fatigue (Blount et al., 2016; Hou & Skovholt, 2020; W. Lee et al., 2014).

Jungbluth et al. (2011) surveyed first- and second-year genetic counseling students about the frequency and intensity of 24 professional and personal stressors. Table 12.1 lists 8 of their most highly ranked stressors in terms of frequency and intensity. Students reported experiencing a mixture of professional/academic and personal stressors. Some stressors were highly problematic regardless of their frequency. For instance, relationship difficulties is a stressor that ranked 12th in frequency but 6th in terms of intensity.

Supervisor Responsibilities

Supervisors should offer guidance and support to students around wellness and self-care, especially as they pertain to challenging aspects of genetic counseling practice and genetic counseling supervision. Supervisor modeling and discussion of self-care can normalize this practice and emphasize the value of wellness to students. For example, emotional aspects of genetic counseling cases pose a major professional challenge to wellness. Included among the genetic counseling supervisor competencies identified by Eubanks Higgins et al. (2013) is helping students process and learn effective coping strategies

TABLE 12.1 Genetic Counseling Students' Most Frequent Stressors and Their Intensity

Stressor	Frequency Ranking	Intensity Ranking[a]
Academic coursework	1	2
Financial strain	2	1
Lack of recreation	3	3
School performance	4	5
Commuting	5	7
Sleeping difficulties	6	4
Change in residence	7	12
Interactions with supervisors/faculty	8	8

[a] Intensity was defined as how problematic the stressor is.

Source: Data from Jungbluth, C., MacFarlane, I. M., McCarthy Veach, P., & LeRoy, B. S. (2011). Why is everyone so anxious? An exploration of stress and anxiety in genetic counseling graduate students. *Journal of Genetic Counseling, 20*, 270–286.

for emotionally difficult cases. Students encounter additional professional challenges related to dealing with their feelings and thoughts about counseling with a supervisor present during sessions and being evaluated on all aspects of their performance (Barnett & Molzon, 2014). The Reciprocal-Engagement Model of Supervision states that supervisors should address student feelings about and responses to supervision and genetic counseling (Wherley et al., 2015).

Howard (2008) asserts that supervisors have a responsibility to not only address student skill development and ethical and professional behavior but also provide support related to their well-being and the emotional effects of clinical work. She further states that the extent to which each of these areas is the focus depends on a student's needs at a given time.

Blount et al. (2016) interviewed clinical mental health supervisors about their experiences around supervisee wellness. They found five themes:

Self-care: Supervisors expressed a belief that taking care of one-self is necessary before being able to care for others.

Intentionality: The supervisors deliberately used strategies to pro-mote their supervisees' self-awareness and understanding of themselves and their clients. Strategies included discussion about wellness and also supervisor modeling of wellness.

Humanness: Both supervisee and supervisor culture, history, background, and prior life experiences influence their current views and behaviors in counseling and supervision. In the absence of reflection and self-awareness, these factors may cause "unintentional blindness" in counseling and supervision relationships.

Support: Supervisors stressed that significant professional and personal relationships are critical aspects of wellness. They further noted that "separating personal life and pro-fessional life aids the supervisor and supervisee in leaving client cases at work and enjoying life beyond the role as a counselor" (p. 368).

Wellness identity: Wellness should be a strong aspect of who a counselor is because it encourages continuous self-reflection on how external factors affect their practice.

Wellness and self-care as they relate to personal issues do not usu-ally take center stage in genetic counseling supervision. Sometimes, however, situations arise outside of the rotation that require attention when they have practice and supervision implications (e.g., a stu-dent has a sudden and unexpected medical emergency or a student experiences the diagnosis of cancer in a family member that makes it more difficult in the short term for them to see clients with cancer).

Whenever you address professional or personal wellness, self-care, and stress/distress with students, you promote their well-being and resilience in the immediate situation and you set the stage for "career-long habits and behaviors" (Barnett & Molzon, 2014, p. 1057). Although wellness and self-care discussions typically occur less frequently in genetic counseling supervision, it is important to pay attention to how your student seems to be functioning (emotionally, cognitively, and physically) and intervene if you have concerns. If you do not feel you have the context or resources to intervene, you should contact the student's graduate program for assistance in assessing and supporting the student's wellness needs.

Wellness and Self-Care Strategies

The following sections describe a variety of strategies, some that are better suited to genetic counseling program professional development activities and others that are relevant for individual supervision relationships. The strategies vary in their depth and the time involved. I suggest you review each strategy to identify those that are feasible for your situation.

General Strategies

Venart et al. (2007) describe numerous wellness strategies that align with Myers et al.'s (2000) wellness domains. The following strategies address four of those domains (pp. 52–59):

Physical wellness strategies
- Get enough sleep, nutrition, and physical activity. Fatigued and physically depleted individuals are at much higher risk of becoming ill, making poor decisions, and reacting impulsively.
- Use strategies to calm the body such as monitoring and deepening your breathing throughout the workday, meditation, massage, and progressive muscle relaxation.

- Ground yourself by paying attention to bodily signals [including during genetic counseling sessions and supervision meetings]. Throughout the day listen to internal cues (e.g., Am I tired? Stressed? Hungry? Lonely?).

Emotional wellness strategies
- Try to tune into feelings. Avoid denying or minimizing feelings. Clues that avoidance is occurring include engaging in escapist activities (e.g., computer games, drinking, surfing the internet). Instead, spend quiet time alone, engage in conversation, watch an inspiring film, read a good article or book, play with a pet, spend some time on a hobby.
- Practice self-reflection. Think about your genetic counseling work and accompanying emotional reactions.
- Express emotions. Research shows journaling (writing about or recording) one's deepest thoughts and feelings can be restorative and improve academic and fieldwork performance.

Cognitive wellness strategies
- Cultivate healthy thinking patterns by recognizing and avoiding catastrophic and all or nothing thinking and noticing small victories.
- Acknowledge what you do not know, admit mistakes, and give yourself credit for what you know and do correctly.
- Remain curious rather than fearful of new and/or ambiguous situations.
- Savor and celebrate small victories in your professional development.

Interpersonal wellness strategies
- Social support is one of the strongest predictors of positive mental health functioning across the life span.
  - Spend time with family and friends, especially those who provide a high quality of support.
  - Consider personal therapy for reducing physical and emotional distress.
  - Seek peer consultation/supervision/support.

Genetic counseling programs could share these strategies with students during professional development meetings. Individual supervisors could suggest the strategies to students who are struggling with wellness in one or more domain.

Genetic Counselor Wellness Strategies

Miranda et al. (2016) asked master genetic counselors how they cope with the emotional intensity of genetic counseling work. Participants identified several coping strategies that align with self-care and wellness. Strategies included setting boundaries around their emotional investment and separating their professional and personal lives by

> compartmentalizing or implementing an "off-switch" (e.g., "I can go home and say it's awful what these folks are dealing with, but it doesn't emotionally tear at me. I think I've learned, or forced myself to compartmentalize, and work is work, and home is home"). (p. 779)

Additional coping strategies included drawing strength/support from loved ones, self-reflection, physical activity, and journaling. Some counselors identified how important it is to allow themselves to experience their feelings: " 'Sometimes I just go with whatever I'm feeling. If something is following me home, if I'm feeling sad, I just need the space to kind of dwell on it a little bit. I may not try to dispel it' " (p. 779). Other counselors used cognitive strategies such as developing a philosophical view that allowed them to accept their limitations and recognizing that certain challenges are intrinsic to genetic counseling.

Strategies that encourage wellness are unique to each genetic counselor practitioner and student, and multiple strategies may be more effective than a single approach (Werner-Lin et al., 2016).

Specific Strategies

A variety of cognitive and behavioral strategies may be effective for helping students manage stress and generally maintain wellness. They contain elements of Baker's (2003) three self-care components (self-awareness, self-regulation, and balance) and resilience characteristics described previously in this chapter (Hou & Skovholt, 2020).

Practice and Model Wellness

Supervisor "best practices" include modeling self-care for students (Borders, 2014). Make efforts to maintain your own wellness, including balancing your personal and professional lives (Barnett & Molzon, 2014). As Lenz and Smith (2010) note,

> It is important that supervisors are committed to wellness development in themselves as well as in supervisees and clients. The mantra behind this contention is adequately noted in the aphorism "Be the change you want to see in the world." (p. 241)

Create an Expectation That Wellness and Self-Care Matter

As often is the case, it is one thing to know that self-care is important, but it is another to implement it.
—BAKER (2003, P. 18)

Engage your student in discussion of wellness and self-care as a right and a professional responsibility of genetic counselors. Cognitively reframe student misperceptions. For instance, state that self-care is not "selfish," it is a necessity. Challenge mistaken beliefs that self-care is too much trouble and/or takes too much time, "as professionals and as human beings, [we] have the right, and deserve, to share with ourselves the same time, care, and tenderness we extend to clients, family and friends" (Baker, 2003, p. 18). Anticipating and initiating discussion of students' mistaken ideas about self-care has an added benefit of modeling "ways for students to anticipate and address difficult patient issues and emotions" (Wherley et al., 2015, p. 712).

Be Systematic

Lenz and Smith (2010) suggest several supervision processes and associated strategies to promote student wellness. These may be utilized by individual supervisors or, more likely, by genetic counseling graduate programs:

> *Education.* Ask students how they define wellness. One option is to ask them to write for 5 minutes about their definition and also what wellness personally looks like for them and to share their description with you. Offer wellness resources and/or present a model of wellness (e.g., Myers et al.'s [2000] Wheel of Wellness model). Many strategies for promoting wellness and self-care exist and are available in books and through the internet. You may want to suggest students make use of some.

> *Assessment.* Ask students to gauge their wellness (e.g., through self-reflection or journaling) and share your assessment/impressions of their functioning, as appropriate. Engage in periodic assessment during your supervision relationship. Strategies can involve both informal and formal conversations and/or use of a brief oral or written scale. For instance, students could "rate their present level of wellness, their personal satisfaction, and their desired level of a particular wellness variable using a 10-point scale [1 = low, 10 = high]" (Lenz & Smith, 2010, p. 238).

> *Planning.* Ask students to identify an aspect of wellness they would like to improve. Inform them that positive change in one area often contributes to overall wellness.

Evaluation. Approximately once each week, briefly check in as to their progress. You may wish to suggest they keep a wellness journal to note their progress.

Caveats. In the planning process, caution students to limit themselves to one wellness domain and one or two aspects within the domain so they do not become overwhelmed (e.g., eat well-balanced meals [physical domain]). Encourage them to select a goal that reflects something they *want* to work on and not something they think they *should* address. Importantly, inform students that their progress or lack thereof on the goal is *not* part of their rotation evaluation. Relatedly, some students may believe that discussions of their overall wellness are outside of the boundary of the supervision relationship. Thus, discussion of privacy, boundaries, and confidentiality may be particularly important for how you approach wellness within supervision.

Encourage Self-Reflective Practice

Almost everything will work again if you unplug it for a few minutes, including you.

—ANNE LAMOTT (ANQUOTES, N.D.)

Self-reflective practice is an introspective strategy for promoting wellness (Orchowski et al., 2010; see also Chapter 9, this volume). Ask your student to maintain a journal in which they reflect on topics you/they consider important during the rotation. Suggest that, for 1 week, they focus on wellness. As Bannink (2006) recommends, ask them to

> pay attention to the things in your life that you would like to keep the way they are and write them down. Pay a compliment to yourself at the end of every day based on the goals written in your ... [journal] and write it down as well. (p. 12)

You could ask them to do one entry for things in their personal life and one for things in their professional life.

Decide whether you wish to review your student's journal entries. A potential benefit is providing insight into their functioning. A potential drawback is impression management—that is, they will write what they think you want to hear.

Other introspective strategies also promote self-reflection. Werner-Lin et al. (2016) suggested "engaging in contemplative practices such as mindfulness will allow the counselor to monitor her own feelings, biases, and assumptions to permit self-acceptance while also enhancing patient care" (p. 865). Mindfulness is a type of meditative practice in which individuals bring their attention to the present moment without judgment of the thoughts, feelings, and physical sensations they are experiencing. You can encourage students to browse the internet for mindfulness practice instructions.

Use Stress Management Strategies

Discuss stressful events or issues related to genetic counseling, monitor your student's workload, and provide support and guidance to assist them in debriefing their feelings after difficult situations (Howard, 2008). The following are questions you could ask a student to reduce their distress and build self-efficacy (Howard, 2008):

> How have you managed in these situations before? What strengths have you drawn on in your past life that might be useful here? What in your experience tells you that you will be able to achieve this? How can you remind yourself of your competence when you are faced with a difficult situation? (p. 110)

Note that the first two questions parallel the types of questions genetic counselors ask clients about their coping and decision-making.

Encourage your student to use a brief self-care strategy prior to each genetic counseling session, when feasible. For example, they could do a 1-minute visualization as follows: Select a calming scene of your choice (walking in a summer meadow, floating down a gently flowing river, etc.); close your eyes, breathe regularly, and for 1 minute imagine yourself in that scene. Another strategy is to visualize themself putting their daily concerns into a drawer and shutting the drawer, recognizing they can open the drawer and retrieve their concerns at some point after the genetic counseling session. Brief physical exercises may also be helpful—for example, placing their hand on their diaphragm and paying attention to their breathing as they inhale and exhale for 30–60 seconds. These are calming strategies that may help students come to sessions with a better focus on the clients.

Assign a Wellness Self-Report Scale

Ask your student to complete a brief scale at least one time during the rotation to allow them to consider different aspects of their functioning. The Self-Care Behavioral Inventory (Santana & Fouad, 2017; see Appendix 12A) is a 19-item measure that assesses professional and personal self-care. I suggest you not require students to share their answers with you, although some may voluntarily do so. Assure them their responses to this scale will not be part of their evaluation.

Tips for Promoting Student Self-Care Practices

Baker (2003) offers several suggestions that you might recommend to students to guide their self-care activities:

- Build in "self-time" at different points during the day to engage in self-care.
- Do things that are relaxing and restorative.

- When selecting activities that assist in coping with stress/distress, avoid those that carry a heavy cost (e.g., isolation and overindulgence in food or alcohol).
- Develop healthy stress-releasing actions.
- Practice self-compassion and self-acceptance.

I further suggest encouraging students to be realistic—it is not possible to meet self-care goals "perfectly." Moreover, when self-care is a "should" rather than a "want," it may become another stressor, which defeats the purpose. Finally, given busy schedules, tight budgets, and so forth, encourage students to think creatively about self-care activities that are quick and/or affordable.

Closing Thoughts

Self-care is not a waste of time; self-care makes your use of time more sustainable.
—JACKIE VIRAMONTEZ (ANQUOTES, N.D.)

Wellness is a dynamic state that requires ongoing attention. It is difficult, if not impossible, to maintain equal balance across all wellness domains. Furthermore, we sometimes "neglect" a certain wellness area(s) in order to accomplish other desired goals. Large imbalances, however, should not become a way of life. Self-care strategies play a powerful role in maintaining wellness. They do not have to be expensive, complex, or time-consuming. Small efforts can make a noticeable difference.

Learning Activities

Most learning activities can be adapted for dyad or small group discussions or for written exercises. Time estimates are provided for discussions, but additional time should be allotted for large group processing.

Activity 12.1 Self-Care Practices

In small groups, discuss the following questions:

Part I: Self-reflection
- How do you define self-care?
- What are your personal self-care needs?
- What are your professional self-care needs?
- How do you practice self-care (in and outside the clinic)?
- How does it feel to think of self-care as a right?
- What are three activities that could be self-care for you?

Part II: Student self-care
- What do you think are barriers to students engaging in self-care?
- What are five professional self-care things students could do that take less than 15 minutes and cost little or nothing?
- What are five personal self-care things students could do that take less than 15 minutes and cost little or nothing?

Estimated time: 40–45 minutes for both parts

Activity 12.2 Assessing Student Wellness

With a partner or in small groups:

- List five or six questions you could ask a student to assess their current wellness. In formulating the questions, consider ones that are not overly intrusive.
- Share your list with the larger group.

Estimated time: 25 minutes

Note: Participants could be asked to list questions for Myers et al.'s (2000) wellness domains.

Activity 12.3 Setting Wellness Goals

- Select a wellness domain (physical, emotional, etc.) as a goal you wish to work on. Limit yourself to one or two aspects of the domain.
- List simple steps for working on your goal. [*Hint*: You could create a mind map, described in Chapter 6, to list the steps.]
- Share your steps with a partner.

Estimated time: 15 minutes

Activity 12.4 Sources of Stress and Stress Management

Part I: Personal Stress Levels

With a partner or in small groups, discuss the following:

- When you were (or as you are) training to be a genetic counselor, what things caused you stress? Why?
- How much of your stress came (or comes) from within yourself versus outside yourself?
- What did (or do) you do to manage your stress? Which of these strategies were/are effective?

Part II: Assessing Student Stress Levels

With a partner or in small groups:

- List specific strategies you could use to gauge students' stress level.
- Include specific questions you might ask students to gauge their stress level.

Estimated time: 30 minutes for both parts

Note: Part II could be expanded to include creating a brief stress assessment form for students to complete.

Activity 12.5 Self-Care Behavior

Individually complete the Self-Care Behavior Inventory (Santana & Fouad, 2017) contained in Appendix 12A.

With a partner or in small groups, share some of your responses to the inventory.

Estimated time: 20–25 minutes

Appendix 12A
Self-Care Behavior Inventory

Rate the frequency of your engagement (or not) in each of the following practices:

	1 Never	2 Rarely	3 Sometimes	4 Most of the time	5 Always
1. Spend time with others you enjoy	___	___	___	___	___
2. Maintain deep interpersonal relationships	___	___	___	___	___
3. Stay in contact with important people	___	___	___	___	___
4. Seek out projects that are exciting or rewarding	___	___	___	___	___
5. Take time to chat with peers	___	___	___	___	___
6. Allow yourself to laugh	___	___	___	___	___
7. Quiet time to complete tasks	___	___	___	___	___
8. Seek out comforting activities	___	___	___	___	___
9. Be open to not knowing	___	___	___	___	___
10. Eat healthy	___	___	___	___	___
11. Exercise	___	___	___	___	___
12. Spend time in nature	___	___	___	___	___
13. Medical care	___	___	___	___	___

14. Take vacations   ___ ___   ___   ___   ___
15. Time off   ___ ___   ___   ___   ___
16. Pray/meditate   ___ ___   ___   ___   ___
17. Connect with spirituality   ___ ___   ___   ___   ___
18. Contribute to causes   ___ ___   ___   ___   ___
19. Advocate   ___ ___   ___   ___   ___

Factor I (Items 1–9): Cognitive–Emotional–Relational
Factor II (Items 10–15): Physical
Factor III (Items 16–19): Spiritual

Note: There are no cutoff scores for this inventory, as each person may differ in how often they need to engage in self-care behaviors to maintain functioning.

Source: Santana, M. C., & Fouad, N. A. (2017). Development and validation of a Self-Care Behavior Inventory. *Training and Education in Professional Psychology, 11*, 140–145. Reprinted with permission from *Training and Education in Professional Psychology*.

13

Recognizing and Addressing Student Problematic Performance

PATRICIA MCCARTHY VEACH

Objectives

- Define problematic performance and its sources.
- Identify cues that student performance is problematic.
- Describe methods to address problematic performance.

How can I not feel guilty when I have to tell a student that they're doing a bad job?

—GENETIC COUNSELING SUPERVISOR

One of the most distressing supervision situations for all involved parties occurs when a student's performance is problematic and not easily resolved. Falendar et al. (2009) note,

> Supervisors must balance responsibilities to ensure client care, facilitate professional development, provide meaningful feedback, and serve as gatekeepers while working to establish and sustain an effective supervisory alliance. This balancing act becomes particularly challenging when supervisors observe problematic behavior or standard performance that requires management. (p. 240)

Genetic counseling supervisor competencies include four remediation activities (Eubanks Higgins et al., 2013; see also Chapter 1, Appendix 1A):

- Recognize student impairment and take steps to document if needed.
- Interact with genetic counseling program faculty to discuss difficulties with students.
- As needed, collaborate with genetic counseling program faculty to create for students with impairment interventions relevant to areas of deficit.
- As needed, provide information about consequences of underperformance.

Problematic performance ranges in severity, and remediation actions vary accordingly. Historically, genetic counseling student problematic performance that requires extreme actions (e.g., dismissal from a program) has been rare. When problematic performance occurs, it is critical that supervisors give students opportunities for remediation and take "necessary action to prevent continued progression toward independent practice in the profession if remediation is not successful" (Barnett & Molzon, 2014, p. 1055).

What Is Problematic Performance?

Problematic performance is "a broad term, encompassing diminished professional functioning attributable to any of the following:

- personal distress, burnout, and/or substance abuse,
- unethical professional behavior, and
- incompetent professional behavior" (Forrest et al.,1999, pp. 631–632).

Student performance may best be conceptualized on a continuum, with problematic functioning at one end and developmental ("not unexpected or excessive" [Lamb et al., 1991, p. 292]) functioning at the other end. Falendar et al. (2009) state,

> Although there is no absolute litmus test for problematic behavior, violations of ethical, professional, and legal standards . . .[behaviors] that pose a risk to client welfare, or the inability to meet a minimum level of competence to perform the responsibilities of the training rotation, are distinct from normal developmental challenges. (p. 243)

The closer a student's functioning comes to the problematic side of the continuum, the more necessary it will be for you to begin remediation efforts.

Problematic Performance Indicators

Reflection Question for Readers: What are two indicators that suggest to you a student is heading toward problematic performance?

A student's behaviors are likely to be problematic when most of the following are present:

- The problem is *pervasive*—that is, not restricted to one area of functioning (Lamb et al., 1991, p. 292).
- The student displays *low awareness* of the problem.
- The student is *nonresponsive*, failing to acknowledge, understand, or address the problem once it is identified (Lamb et al., 1991, p. 292).
- *Chronicity and depth* of the problem are extensive.
- The problem has a *deleterious effect* on
  - genetic counseling services, and/or
  - supervision.
- The quality of services provided by the student is *consistently negatively affected* (Lamb et al., 1991, p. 292).

- The problem is *not quickly or easily rectified.*
- The behavior(s) associated with the problem seems to be *relatively permanent.* The behavior(s) does not change with feedback, remediation efforts, and/or time (Lamb et al., 1991, p. 292).
- Supervisors and other training personnel are giving a *disproportionate amount of attention* to the problem (Lamb et al., 1991, p. 292).

Types of Problematic Performance

Clinical Competence Domains

Overholser and Fine (1990) identified five domains of problematic performance around clinical competence:

> *Lack of factual knowledge*: Lack of knowledge includes possessing an inadequate knowledge base and/or an inability to recognize the limitations of one's knowledge and expertise.
>
> *Example*: Student unknowingly provides clients incorrect information about genetic testing options.
>
> *Deficient technical skills*: Lack of technical skills refers to an inability to correctly use special techniques or procedures in the clinical setting.
>
> *Example*: Student is unable to perform an appropriate risk analysis for hereditary cancer.
>
> *Poor judgment*: Poor judgment involves an inability to select and apply knowledge and skills necessary to plan for and counsel a given client. Instead, the student uses generic approaches for all clients.
>
> *Example*: Student gives detailed explanations using scientific jargon to clients who have limited cognitive abilities.
>
> *Disturbing interpersonal attributes*: Disturbing interpersonal attributes consist of personality characteristics, social skills, and emotional problems affecting professional functioning.

Note some aspects of these attributes are modifiable, whereas others are less so.

Example: Student is highly emotional when discussing abnormal test results with clients.

Inadequate generic clinical skills: Inadequate clinical skills involve a lack of basic helping skills necessary to accurately assess and respond to clients, such as empathy, warmth, genuineness, questioning skills, and awareness of how their own characteristics affect session processes and outcomes.

Example: Student fails to recognize and acknowledge clients' emotional reactions.

Diminished Functioning Versus Unsuitability

Veilleux et al. (2012) studied perceptions of diminished functioning and unsuitability in clinical psychology graduate students. The researchers defined *diminished functioning* as referring to students who may have previously functioned at a competent level or showed potential for competent behavior but are dealing with situational issues (e.g., life stressors) that affect their performance. They defined *unsuitability* as referring to students whose performance suggests they "lack the capacity" for their professional career (Veilleux et al., 2012). They identified three factors related to diminished functioning and unsuitability (p. 117):

Trait characteristics: Trait characteristics are "longstanding internal character deficits" (p. 117). Examples include immaturity, lack of self-awareness, lack of interpersonal skills, lack of communication skills, and lack of intellectual reasoning. Inherent characteristics may or may not be teachable skills.

General distress: General distress includes transient (acute) stress-related issues such as anxiety, physical illness, financial strain, major life changes, and depression. Given their temporal nature, they may be more easily resolved.

318 | CLINICAL SUPERVISION IN GENETIC COUNSELING

Chronic pathology: Chronic pathology involves habitual "externalizing" of psychological conditions and includes alcohol abuse/dependence, drug abuse/dependence, personality disorder, and anger management. These issues vary with respect to being modifiable.

It is important to acknowledge the subjectivity of these assessments. Subjectivity may arise from individual supervisor factors (e.g., countertransference; see Chapter 14) and/or systemic factors (e.g., current and historic institutionalized racism in both health care and higher education). For these reasons, supervisors need to pay particular attention to whether personal, cultural, or other biases are affecting their judgment of these categories.

Addressing Problematic Performance

Addressing problematic performance is a particularly challenging aspect of supervision (Russell et al., 2007). Falendar et al. (2009) state that "after ensuring client care (their first responsibility), supervisors enter into processes in which they must articulate specific areas of problematic professional behavior and develop with their supervisees plans to enhance clinical competence" (p. 247). Within these processes, supervisors must distinguish between "developmentally normative" difficulties and those that require a more remedial approach (Falendar et al., 2009). In genetic counseling, it is critical for supervisors to remember that the graduate program is ultimately responsible for students' behavior. Any action taken to address problematic behavior *must occur in collaboration* with the student's program.

Student performance that would require remediation includes "an inability to achieve an appropriate level of competence after sufficient training and supervision, lapses in capability ... [and/or] significant lapses in professional judgment and failures to adhere to professional, ethical, and legal standards"

(Falendar et al., 2009, p. 240). Supervisors should address such performance directly and soon (Russell et al., 2007). As Barnett and Molzon (2014) state,

> It may be tempting to take a "wait and see" approach, but if . . . consecutive supervisors take this approach, a supervisee with inadequate clinical skills or who does not possess the needed personality attributes or disposition may be passed along . . . to the likely detriment of future clients and . . . the profession. (pp. 1054–1055)

Several strategies, described next, offer guidance for responding to problematic performance.

Identify Barriers to Addressing Student Behaviors

Reflection Question for Readers: Can you think of reasons that you, personally, might wish to avoid addressing a student's problematic behaviors?

Several factors might make a supervisor hesitant to take on difficult behaviors (Forrest et al., 1999, pp. 646–647):

Disagreement: Not everyone agrees about what behaviors constitute inadequate performance.

Subjectivity: Judgments about a student's personal attributes (e.g., maturity level) seem more subjective than other types of judgments (e.g., accuracy in calculating a risk rate).

Ambivalence: The supervisor feels torn between evaluating and nurturing.

Lack of information: The student may withhold critical information that would clarify the scope of their behavior.

Reprisal: The supervisor fears an adversarial and time-consuming process, with the potential for litigation.

Privacy: The supervisor wishes to protect the student's privacy.

Long-range consequences: The supervisor is concerned about the implications for the student's career and well-being.

Wishful thinking: The supervisor hopes the problem will self-correct over time.

Additional barriers involve wondering whether the student's behavior is a reflection of one's skills as a supervisor; and cognitive dissonance given the student's prior strong performance in courses and rotations.

Try to identify which of these factors may pose barriers for you (e.g., consult with a peer). Work to set them aside in order to move forward.

Follow a Deliberate Process

When you think a student's performance is problematic, take the following steps: report, review, document, and remediate. Throughout this four-step process, consult and work with other relevant parties as warranted (e.g., other supervisors at your site, administrators, and program faculty).

Report

When you have decided that a student's performance is problematic, report your concerns to the student's genetic counseling program director or other designated program leadership responsible for clinical training. In collaboration with the program, develop a plan for addressing this behavior.

Review

Once you decide the student's performance is problematic rather than a typical developmental issue, ask yourself these questions (Lamb et al., 1991, p. 293):

- What specific behaviors are concerning, and are they included in the overall evaluation criteria?
- How and in what situations has the student demonstrated these behaviors?
- Who has observed the behaviors?
- Who or what was affected by the behaviors (clients, training program, clinic atmosphere, etc.)?
- How frequent are the behaviors?
- Has the student been made aware of these behaviors, and if so, how did they respond?
- Have I documented my feedback about their behavior in any way?
- How serious are their behaviors on a continuum of ethical and professional functioning?

Document

Lawyers will say if something isn't written, it didn't happen. Write down your responses to the questions in the previous section. Keep notes about conversations and meetings with the student and other involved parties and the dates of those conversations. Write down the names of individuals with whom you consulted and the dates of those consultations. Accurate and complete documentation is especially critical for situations in which you are unable to reach a mutual understanding with the student about their problematic performance and/or how to remediate it (Russell et al., 2007). Share all documentation with the student's graduate program director because ultimately assessment of remediation and decisions about student progress or dismissal will fall to the program.

Remediate

Decide upon and implement actions to respond to the student's problematic performance in collaboration with the genetic counseling program director. Russell et al. (2007) studied marriage and family therapy supervisors and found they preferred to initially respond with "less severe actions, such as talking to the student or consulting with other faculty, before implementing more severe consequences" (p. 235). They commonly considered two factors when choosing how to respond: whether the student's behavior or problem occurred for the first time or had been addressed before, and whether it posed possible risks to clients. Some supervisors also mentioned the importance of considering a student's culture (e.g., regarding issues such as physical contact). Participants identified several possible actions that the Russell et al. grouped into six categories (p. 232):

Talk: Have a conversation with the student; discuss with faculty.

Referral: Refer student for psychological assessment; refer for personal therapy.

Begin due process: Write a letter of concern; create a remediation plan.

Increase interaction: Provide more supervision; require the student to repeat specific courses or rotation(s); increase informal communication with the student.

Mutual gatekeeping: Give the student a leave of absence; counsel them out of the program.

Unilateral gatekeeping: Place the student on probation; dismiss student from the rotation or the program.

The specific actions taken should depend on the nature of the problematic performance. More egregious behavior and behaviors indicative of unsuitability for the genetic counseling profession require stronger remediation actions based on input from all relevant parties (e.g., supervisor or supervisors, the student's program faculty, and clinic administrators). Remediation plans should include specific milestones that will indicate a student's performance is back on track and meeting expectations. Note that when you identify any type of student behavior suggesting a need for remediation, you should inform the student's program director *as soon as possible*. In most situations, implementation of the six categories listed above will be done by (or in collaboration with) leadership of the student's graduate program.

I cannot stress enough how essential it is for you to inform program leadership when there is a problem; if you remain silent, they will not know and will not be able to address the issue. I also remind you that aspects of a student's problematic performance are sometimes confidential and therefore program leaders may be unable to share certain information and/or remediation efforts with you. In these situations, do not assume that program faculty have "done nothing."

Prepare Yourself for Initial Conversations

Engaging in conversations with relevant parties is a crucial part of remediation. Conversations are necessary when normal formative and summative feedback to a student has been ineffective or when new problematic behaviors arise (Jacobs et al., 2011). One of these conversations should take place between you and the student to specify and discuss the behavior and why it is problematic (Falendar et al. 2009).

These conversations can be challenging for several reasons. For instance, you may have had limited guidance about how to conceptualize and address student "problems"; defining specific behaviors that are concerning is not simple; speaking about performance issues with a student or other colleagues can be painful; and/or you worry about the student taking a self-protective stance (e.g., denying, arguing, and crying) (Jacobs et al., 2011). There are several things you can do to ready yourself for difficult conversations:

- Self-reflect. What are your experience, comfort, and skills for addressing certain student competencies? Ask yourself how you feel about the student's behavior (anxious, hopeless, angry, etc.) (Jacobs et al., 2011). Use Lamb et al.'s (1991) criteria, described previously in this chapter, to support your assessment of problematic performance.

- Consult with colleagues. What are you most concerned about? What would be a positive outcome of remediation attempts? Is the problematic performance due to the student's personal characteristics, environmental factors (e.g., stressors), or interaction between the two? Do you think the student's performance can improve, or is it fairly permanent? Russell et al. (2007) note that three "bottom line" questions may help you balance the needs of students with those of other stakeholders. Ask yourself "(1) Would I be comfortable hiring this person? (2) Would I be willing to supervise this person as my employee? (3) Would I refer a family member to this [person]?" (p. 239). Consultation will help you recognize any tendency to either over-interpret behavior as problematic or discount problematic behavior as "typical." Remember to ensure student confidentiality and privacy when consulting with others.

- Limit discussion to those individuals who have a need to know. Do not discuss a student's issues with other students or with genetic counselors outside of your site.

- Notify the student's program director. Problematic performance issues require you to inform the student's program leadership and to do so as soon as possible. Depending on the nature and severity of the issue, program leadership may want to meet with you and other relevant parties to begin a remediation plan prior to and/or after your initial conversation with the student.

- Consult with other experts as needed (e.g., legal and psychological).

- Gather necessary information to address the issue (Jacobs et al., 2011).

- Prepare "talking points" based on established competency domains and a developmentally expected performance level. I strongly suggest you avoid using the terms *impaired* and *impairment* (despite their use in Eubanks Higgins et al.'s

[2013] supervisor competencies) because "in addition to being an imprecise, and perhaps misleading, shorthand method of communicating performance deficiencies, use of these terms raises serious legal issues under the ADA [Americans with Disabilities Act]" (Falender et al., 2009, p. 241; Falender et al. provide an in-depth discussion of this issue).

- Practice with colleagues what you will say to the student (Jacobs et al., 2011).
- Anticipate how the student is likely to respond (distress, argumentativeness, silence, etc.) (Jacobs et al., 2011).

Be Planful and Deliberate During Conversations

- Arrange a private space for the conversation.
- Schedule sufficient time to discuss the issue with your student.
- Recognize that it is natural for both you and your student to feel anxious.
- Move directly to the topic. Do not avoid the issue by engaging in unrelated discussion.
- Use your talking points to frame the conversation.
- Be sensitive to the emotional impact of your words (Jacobs et al., 2011), and strike a balance between being overly blunt and vague.
- Describe the behavior—give specific examples.
- Point out clinical ramifications of the behavior.
- Ask your student what they are thinking and feeling during the conversation. If they seem highly defensive, consider giving them some time to process what they are hearing before proceeding (e.g., a quick break or later in the day) (Jacobs et al., 2011). Tell your student (and remind yourself) that the conversation and possible action plan are not intended as a punishment; they are to ensure a standard of care for clients and to support the student's well-being.
- Use a problem-solving approach. Ask your student, "Do you think you can achieve behavioral expectations? If so, how

might you do that? How might I help in that process?" (Jacobs et al., 2011).

- Inform your student of likely next steps (student actions, your actions, and other relevant parties' actions).
- Ask your student to verbally summarize the major points of the conversation. Clarify any misperceptions.
- Document the conversation.
- Document future conversation(s) and note student progress on identified competencies of concern (Jacobs et al., 2011).
- Share documentation with the student's genetic counseling program leadership.

Additional Strategies to Support Remediation Efforts

Use a Supervision Agreement

A supervision agreement (see Chapter 3), presented and discussed at the beginning of supervision, will include clear expectations about student performance and student and supervisor responsibilities around expected performance (Russell et al., 2007).

Follow Clinic Policy

Use your site's policies and procedures that support remediation plans for student problematic performance (Jacobs et al., 2011). If your site does not have these types of policies, I encourage you to work toward their development.

Review Genetic Counseling Program Policies

Programs accredited by the Accreditation Council for Genetic Counseling are required to include a policy in their student handbook about addressing student problematic performance. The policy should include guidelines about confidentiality boundaries regarding student performance so supervisors and students know what communications will occur among supervisors/faculty and what will be shared with students.

Participate in Peer Supervision

Peer supervision (see Chapter 15) can provide support and guidance around confidential discussions of challenging supervision situations, including student problematic performance.

Closing Thoughts

As Overholser (2004) states, "supervision can be a wonderful process for monitoring, evaluating, and collaborating. . . . [Sometimes, however,] supervision is a challenging process that requires patience and persistence" (p. 11). When a student's behavior requires remediation, the challenges may be intense. Given the complexity and distressing nature of problematic performance, you should never try to "go it alone." Everyone (clients, students, colleagues, and you) will benefit from the input of individuals directly involved in the student's professional preparation.

Overholser (2004) offers a gardening analogy for supervision, describing it as "planting seeds that will take time to grow . . . proper growth will need a safe and protective environment, fertile soil, a warm sun, and plenty of water" (p. 11). As with any garden, when it comes to problematic performance, students will need individualized attention and care. Many, although not all, will thrive as a result.

Learning Activities

Most learning activities can be adapted for dyad or small group discussions or for written exercises. Time estimates are provided for discussions, but additional time should be allotted for large group processing.

Activity 13.1 Remediation Conversations

Conversations regarding problematic performance share certain similarities to giving bad news to clients. Prepare a written response to each of these bullet points:

- Think of how you go about *preparing* to give bad news to a client. List the things you do.
- Think about how you actually *communicate* the bad news to a client. List what you generally say and do.
- How do the actions on your list *translate* to difficult conversations with students? How do they *differ*?

Share your responses with a partner or in small groups.

Estimated time: 15 minutes

Activity 13.2 Problematic Performance

In small groups, discuss your views of the following:

- What *personal attributes* do you regard as necessary for a student to become a genetic counselor?
- Which of these personal attributes can be taught?
- What *situational stressors* do you think might lead to a decision to have a student take a leave of absence from a rotation?
- What behaviors would lead you to think a student should be removed from the rotation?
- What behaviors would lead you to think a student should be terminated from their program?
- What cultural factors or biases might impact your answers to the previous questions?

Estimated time: 30 minutes

Note: In processing this activity, ask the following: How much consensus did participants have for each question? Why do they think that is? Do participants notice any themes in responses to each discussion question?

Activity 13.3 Barriers to Supervision

Rank order the following barriers in order of how much they would contribute to your hesitancy to address a student's problematic performance (1 = contributes the most; 10 = contributes the least). Then share your responses with a partner.

___ *Disagreement.* Not everyone agrees about what behaviors constitute inadequate performance.

___ *Subjectivity.* Judgments about a student's personal attributes seem more subjective than other types of judgments (e.g., their accuracy in calculating a risk rate).

___ *Ambivalence.* You feel torn between evaluating and nurturing.

___ *Lack of information.* The student may withhold critical information that would clarify the scope of their behavior.

___ *Reprisal.* You fear an adversarial and time-consuming process, with the potential for litigation.

___ *Privacy.* You wish to protect student privacy.

___ *Long-range consequences.* You are concerned about the implications for the student's career and well-being.

___ *Wishful thinking.* You hope the problem will self-correct over time.

___ *Supervisor skills.* You wonder if the student's behavior reflects on your skills.

___ *Prior performance.* The student has performed strongly in other courses and rotations.

Estimated time: 20 minutes

Activity 13.4 Addressing Student Problematic Performance

Part I: Discussion

In small groups, discuss these questions for each of the following scenarios:

- What is the competency(ies) at issue?
- Does the issue involve unsuitability or diminished functioning?
- What do you think the cause might be (e.g., student trait, situational stressor, both)?
- What are implicit biases that could be impacting your perception?
- What will you say to the student?

Scenario*: Your student, who has demonstrated excellent clinical skills in the past, has recently changed in appearance and behavior, becoming withdrawn, irritable, and less careful about personal hygiene. Although continuing to meet with clients, the student has been missing case conference meetings and finds "reasons" to cut short your supervision time. You express concerns about the changes and these behaviors. The student discloses to you that they had been treated for bipolar disorder but is not currently on medication.

Scenario*: You are supervising a novice student who has an unusually difficult time connecting with clients. You have observed them in several genetic counseling sessions and have pointed out how their low activity level and lack of "presence" in the session make it difficult to engage clients in the process. You have role-played new ways of behaving in sessions, but the feedback has made little difference. The student continues to have difficulty engaging clients.

Scenario: Your student portrays an extremely high level of confidence. During debriefings when asked what they might have done differently in a counseling session, the student typically says, "Nothing, really; I think I did a good job." You do not think their skill level warrants such a high level of confidence. When you attempt to provide feedback, the student routinely interrupts you and appears to be only "half-listening." You have noticed similar behaviors with clients.

Scenario: Your student, who is in their final rotation, frequently shows up to clinic late and unprepared. You have discussed these behaviors with the student, but the behaviors continue. The student says, "I'm overwhelmed with work and I already have a job so I'm focusing less time on clinic."

Estimated time: 30 minutes

*Adapted from Russell, C. S., DuPree, W. J., Beggs, M. A., Peterson, C. M., & Anderson, M. P. (2007). Responding to remediation and gatekeeping challenges in supervision. *Journal of Marital and Family Therapy, 33*, 227–244.

Part II: Role Plays

Triads take turns as supervisor, student, and observer for the scenarios described in Part I. After each role play, the observer and student give feedback to the supervisor about how they addressed the issue with the student.

Estimated time: 40 minutes

Activity 13.5 Developing an Intervention to Improve Student Problematic Performance

In small groups, use the mind mapping strategy (described in Chapter 6) to assist a student in addressing one of the problematic performance issues described in the scenarios in Activity 13.4.

- Name a primary *skill* that is deficient in the student's performance.
- Draw a mind map that includes six steps (actions, resources, and experiences) to help the student develop the skill.

Estimated time: 15 minutes

14

Common Clinical Supervision Challenges

PATRICIA MCCARTHY VEACH

Objectives

- Describe three commonly occurring supervision challenges.
- Identify strategies for recognizing and managing these challenges.

This chapter focuses on three prevalent challenges in genetic counseling supervision: conflict, supervisor countertransference, and student anxiety. When left unaddressed, these challenges can result in diminished student well-being and restricted ability to develop their genetic counseling skills (Grant et al., 2012) and supervisor loss of confidence and burnout. Borders (2014) regards supervisors as engaging in *best practices*, when they

> anticipate some level of conflict in the supervisory relationship and deal with it productively. They also address . . . countertransference in developmentally appropriate ways . . . [and] are on the alert to recognize their own unproductive or harmful influences . . . and how these may be contributing to supervisee anxiety, resistance, and relationship conflict. (p. 155)

This chapter contains several strategies for addressing these challenges. Note that many of the strategies described in other chapters of this book overlap with strategies in this chapter. You may want to refer to the other chapters for more details.

Supervisor–Student Conflict

Conflict is a natural dynamic in all relationships, including supervision. Genetic counseling supervisor competencies (Eubanks Higgins et al., 2013; see also Chapter 1, Appendix 1A) include three conflict resolution activities: Genetic counselor supervisors

- recognize that some level of disagreement is inevitable in supervisory relationships and use key principles of conflict resolution to attend to conflicts that interfere with the supervision process;
- resolve problems with interpersonal dynamics that arise by creating an action plan (to include contact with genetic counseling program faculty as needed); and
- provide students with information about due process when they disagree about feedback or a rotation evaluation (check with other genetic counseling supervisors on site, talk with genetic counseling program faculty, etc.).

Types of Supervision Conflicts

Conflicts may arise in supervision for many reasons, including students perceiving the supervisor as not invested in the supervision relationship, not providing enough supervision, feeling as if the supervisor expects the student to support them, and power struggles (Nelson & Friedlander, 2001). Anecdotally, I am aware of situations in which students perceive the supervisor as too controlling—that is, not allowing them autonomy in their counseling and/or jumping in excessively and taking over counseling sessions; having expectations of the student that are too high, too low, or unclear; providing feedback in a belittling way, providing primarily corrective feedback, giving vague feedback, or withholding corrective feedback until the end of the rotation; failing to recognize and incorporate cultural factors; and having "personality clashes." I am also aware of situations in which supervisors perceive the student to be "checked out," overly confident, "entitled," dismissive of feedback and suggestions, passive, and having "personality clashes." These situations share a common feature: They jeopardize the achievement of supervision goals and genetic counseling goals.

Conflict Management Strategies

Although conflict is uncomfortable for everyone, it is essential to take steps to resolve issues when they arise (Grant et al., 2012). The following strategies may be beneficial:

- Take the initiative to discuss conflicts you are aware of with your student. Given the power differential and evaluative nature of supervision, students are unlikely to raise the issue with you (Gray et al., 2001).
- Normalize that some level of conflict is common in supervision or any working relationship, and acknowledge the power differential in supervision.
- Address conflict before it becomes too counterproductive (McCarthy Veach, 2001).
- Consult with a colleague(s) to help you clarify your thoughts and feelings and to consider how to address the conflict while maintaining student confidentiality (Grant et al., 2012; McCarthy Veach, 2001).
- Place the conflict within a context. Consider whether it is due to typical developmental issues (e.g., a more advanced student who feels ready for greater autonomy or a new supervisor who is unsure of when to allow a student to take

on more counseling responsibility) or administrative issues (e.g., the clinic does not allow students to do any part of a genetic counseling session alone or does not give students access to client medical records for case preparation) (Grant et al., 2012).

- Decide how direct to be by considering the student's nature, developmental level, the quality of your relationship, and the complexity of the conflict (Grant et al., 2012). In a study of supervision difficulties, Grant et al. (2012) found that "generally, a less direct form of confrontation was utilized when the supervisee had a fragile personality, was resistant to supervision, or was a trainee who required more opportunity to explore his or her own solutions" (p. 535).
- When addressing conflict, reinforce the student's strengths (Grant et al., 2012).
- If the conflict is a result of your actions, admit your mistake (Grant et al., 2012).
- Review suggestions for having *difficult conversations* (described in Chapter 13).

Three *anticipatory* strategies can facilitate conflict management:

- Use a supervision agreement (see Chapter 3) that includes due process procedures should the student have concerns about their supervision. Along with this agreement, discuss what each of you can do to resolve a misunderstanding should it occur (McCarthy Veach, 2001).
- You may not be aware of conflict the student is experiencing (Gray et al., 2001). Work to build trust and rapport from the beginning. Periodically, do a "supervision check." Ask your student what has been working well so far and what they wish could be different.
- Speak with genetic counseling program faculty about including conflict management in an orientation session for students who are beginning rotations. Strategies could

include role plays and review of due process procedures (McCarthy Veach, 2001).

Example of Addressing a Conflict: Student Autonomy Versus Imitation

Students wish to conduct sessions "their way," but it often is confusing to patients and doesn't work. Eventually we tell students to conduct the session similar to the way we do in order to become competent in the session. Students are resistant to this, and we feel guilty for making them copy us.

—GENETIC COUNSELING SUPERVISOR

Suggested Strategies

- Inform your student at the beginning of the rotation that you expect every student to pattern their counseling after yours, and as they progress, you will work with them to incorporate more of their own style.
- Ask your student what benefits they can see to imitative learning.
- Provide a rationale for imitative learning based on the need for effective and efficient provision of services to clients. Reassure your student that even when imitating, they will be developing their own style if they reflect upon the ways in which your approach does and does not fit for them.
- Acknowledge their frustration.
- Do not feel guilty. Imitation is an essential step in learning.
- Record yourself counseling a client if feasible, or role play with a colleague. Require your student to watch the recording and reflect on what you do and why you do it.
- Assess whether your student's inefficiency or your own anxiety, impatience, or investment in clients is making you overly cautious about giving the student some autonomy.

- Be honest about issues of right or wrong versus "two rights"—stylistic differences may be acceptable provided the client receives a standard of care.
- Acknowledge when students are ready to become more autonomous, and suggest ways they can begin incorporating some of their own style.

Supervisor Countertransference

There is a great deal of unmapped country within us which would have to be taken into account in an explanation of our gusts and storms.
—GEORGE ELLIOTT (AS CITED IN WINSPEAR, 2010, P. 3)

Information and a skill set are not the only things supervisors bring to the relationship. They also bring their own emotions and prior life experiences. Countertransference "refers to conscious and unconscious emotions, fantasies, behaviors, perceptions, and psychological defenses that the genetic counselor experiences as a response *to any aspect* [emphasis added] of the genetic counseling [or supervision] situation" (Redlinger-Grosse, 2020, p. 154). Countertransference essentially "is the same as [student] transference, but in the opposite direction" (Cerney, 1985, p. 362).

Unmanaged countertransference can have several consequences for a supervisor's work with students, including being emotionally draining, disrupting rapport, causing over-identification that hinders empathy and objectivity, disengagement, and boundary crossings and violations (e.g., Reeder et al., 2017). Thus, countertransference may pose a barrier to achieving supervision goals, hinder student development, create conflict, lead to ethical violations, and affect client care. When recognized and managed appropriately, however, countertransference may provide insights because students sometimes unconsciously present themselves to supervisors as clients present to them, or they adopt their supervisor's attitudes and behaviors with clients (Friedlander et al., 1989; Shulman, 2006).

Genetic counseling supervisor competencies (Eubanks Higgins et al., 2013; see also Chapter 1, Appendix 1A) include supervisors being able to recognize and address transference and countertransference issues in supervision in ways that are productive for the supervision process.

Sources of Supervisor Countertransference

Countertransference tends to arise from perceived similarities and differences with students (e.g., physical appearance, mannerisms, interpersonal style, and cultural identities) and/or supervisor history (e.g., unresolved interpersonal issues, having previously experienced a situation similar to the student or their client, and the student or their client's situation is personally threatening). *Over-identification* occurs when you regard the student or the student's client as "just like me"; *dis-identification* occurs when you view the student or client as "nothing like me" (Watkins, 1985).

Types of Countertransference

Kessler (1992) described two broad types of genetic counselor countertransference. Applied to supervision, they are as follows:

> *Projective identification*: You *mistakenly* believe that what you feel and think matches your student's feelings and thoughts.
> *Example*: "You must have felt sad when the client told you about three miscarriages."
> *Associative identification*: Your student's experience taps into your own issues or experiences, and you begin to focus on your personal thoughts and feelings. You know these are your personal reactions, but you become distracted by them.
> *Example*: Your student's distress about clients challenging their expertise touches on your own "imposter" issues.

Countertransference is sometimes a reaction to your student's transference. For instance, some students are highly dependent on approval and will see you as *all knowing*, which may prompt you to disengage from what you see as their limitless need for support. Your countertransference may also be prompted by your student's genetic counseling situations, such as "a particular type of patient (e.g., terminally ill . . .) and/or by certain genetic counseling situations that 'push your buttons' (e.g., sex selection, presymptomatic testing of minors)" (McCarthy Veach et al., 2018, p. 334).

Supervisor countertransference may also be a more habitual type of reaction toward all or most students. Watkins (1985, pp. 357–358) identified four types:

Overprotective countertransference: You regard some or all students as childlike and in need of great care and protection so, for example, you cushion the feedback you give, worry excessively about them, etc.

Benign countertransference: Due to an extreme need to be liked, or a fear of strong emotions (e.g., anger), you create an atmosphere that is the same across all students and situations (characterized by shallow exploration of their performance and feelings about their development, optimism, limited consideration of corrective feedback or challenging issues, and sometimes excessive chitchat).

Rejecting countertransference: You regard students as dependent and react punitively, becoming cold or aloof, using distancing behaviors either from fear of demands students may place on you or from fear of being responsible for their well-being (e.g., blunt answers, dismissive responses—"That's for you to figure out. I'm not the student here").

Hostile countertransference: You dislike something about your student (e.g., mannerism, attitude, or values). To be as unlike the student as possible, you distance yourself, sometimes harshly (e.g., "I already told you I'm not the one prepping this case"; "As we've *already* discussed, the protocol for this type of client is . . .").

Behaviors That Suggest Countertransference

Countertransference can take many forms ... an itch, a fleeting image, a powerful feeling, a bodily sensation, boredom, an inability to think clearly, dissociation, a momentary lapse of attention, a thought which seems totally unrelated to ... the session, sexual feelings, pride, anger, rage, anxiety, happiness, depression, hopelessness, and many others.

—T. STARK
(PERSONAL COMMUNICATION, FEBRUARY 22, 2002)

Box 14.1 contains examples of different types of feelings, thoughts, and overt actions that may indicate countertransference. These behaviors share several commonalities. They involve either strong emotion or the absence of emotion. They are *out of the ordinary* with respect to the way you typically interact with students. Finally, they differ from expected practice (e.g., other colleagues would question your understanding of the student and/or your behavior).

Strategies to Manage Countertransference

The strategies discussed here will help you recognize and manage countertransference.

Use an Ongoing Self-Reflection Process

Recognizing and managing dynamics such as countertransference require self-awareness and self-reflection. Start by considering your beliefs about countertransference. Box 14.2 contains examples of common misperceptions. Ask yourself if you have any of these beliefs and work on correcting them.

Locate the source(s) of your reactions. Ask yourself, "I wonder why this is so? Why did I have that response to the student? What was behind my response? What was I reacting to when making that response? Was my response really related to helping the student?" Journaling may help you gain insight into your countertransference sources and the ways you express it.

BOX 14.1 Examples of Behaviors Indicating Countertransference

Lose all neutrality and side with or against a student

Treat student punitively during supervision and/or when they are counseling

Feel anger and frustration with student; express hostility toward or about student; argue

Being overly intellectual

Idealizing a student

Act in a submissive way with a student during supervision or when they counsel

Overly responsible for a student

Make more suggestions than usual to a student

Engage in too much self-disclosure; supervision feels like chatting with a friend

Express a need to be respected, appreciated, and loved

Act defensively when supervising

Rush in to solve a student's problem

Behave as if you are "somewhere else"; get sleepy; feel bored; space out

Apathetic toward a student; do not feel any caring about a student

Dread seeing a student

Feel protective of a student

Feel hurt by something a student says or does during supervision

End supervision time early or late; forget a meeting with a student

Experience envy, guilt, or pity for a student

Avoid eye contact when supervising

Forget important details about student's performance when discussing in supervision

Feel smug about how much you have helped a student

Use language such as feeling "hooked" or "had" or "sucked in" by a student

Have dreams/nightmares involving a student

---

*Modified from Hofsess, C. D., & Tracey, T. J. G. (2010). Countertransference as a prototype: The development of a measure. *Journal of Counseling Psychology*, 57, 52–67 (pp. 58–59); and T. Stark (personal communication, February 22, 2002).

BOX 14.2 Countertransference Myths and Realities

Myth: Countertransference is always obvious.
Reality: Countertransference often is subtle.
Myth: Countertransference only happens to certain people.
Reality: Countertransference is a universal phenomenon.
Myth: Countertransference only occurs in long-term relationships.
Reality: Countertransference can occur in any relationship regardless of its length.
Myth: Countertransference is only about negative reactions.
Reality: Countertransference can involve both negative and positive feelings.
Myth: Countertransference takes time to develop.
Reality: Countertransference onset is quick.
Myth: Countertransference means I am unskilled.
Reality: Countertransference affects all supervisors regardless of their skill level.

Work on Decreasing Your Anxiety

Countertransference often arises from a real or perceived threat that causes an individual to feel anxious. Relaxation exercises, deep breathing, meditation, and self-talk (e.g., "I don't have to let this get to me") can be helpful.

Seek Peer Support

Countertransference dynamics "can be difficult to address without an objective third party, because they are at least partially unconscious" (McCarthy Veach, 2001, p. 398). Peer consultations and supervision will allow you to discuss your countertransference with colleagues. Although you do need to rectify behavioral consequences of countertransference (e.g., providing more positive feedback to balance your, up to now, heavy emphasis on corrective feedback), it is generally recommended that you *not* disclose the source of your countertransference to the student (e.g., your over-emphasis on corrective feedback is partly due to being raised by a highly critical parent) (Grant et al., 2012). Support from colleagues will help you maintain appropriate boundaries around self-disclosure of countertransference.

Example of Addressing Countertransference: Disliking a Student

Disliking a student is sometimes (although not always) a countertransferential reaction (Boysen et al., 2022). Boysen et al. (2022) surveyed college teachers from several academic fields and found almost half had experienced intense dislike of one or more students. I think their findings are generalizable to supervision.

The most prevalent reasons for the teachers' feelings were student attitudes, personality traits, and irresponsible and disruptive behaviors. Specific behaviors included disrespectful attitude, entitled attitude, dislikable personality traits (e.g., narcissism and smugness), poor work, complaining or whining, aggressive verbal behavior, disengagement or disinterest in learning, and attempting to manipulate (e.g., flattering and seeking sympathy). For example, "[The student] often challenged me—claiming that . . . he knew more than I did" and "He found me multiple times per day to intrusively and anxiously ask me questions . . . in a somewhat angry way" (Boysen et al., 2022, p. 1).

Strategies to Manage Dislike

Participants in Boysen et al.'s (2022) survey identified two overarching strategies:

- Manage student behavior—They suggested you start by managing the student's behavior. If you can stop/modify it, then your reactions should subside. They also recommended addressing "violations of expectations as soon as they emerge rather than ignoring them in hope that they will resolve on their own" (p. 6).

- Manage your reactions—They noted that "maintaining professionalism, assertiveness, and consulting with peers would be most effective. In contrast, they viewed avoiding the student and overcompensating by being extra nice as least effective" (p. 4). They also recommended reframing the situation, self-care, and empathy.

Student Anxiety

[An ancient Ojibwe Mide said] "In every human being there are two wolves constantly fighting. One is fear, and the other is love." Asked "Which of the wolves won the battle," [his] answer had been: "The one you feed. Always the one you feed."

—KRUEGER (2014, P. 6)

Genetic counseling supervisor competencies include addressing student anxiety. Supervisors should recognize that some student anxiety is normal and seek to lessen students' anxieties and help students find productive ways to manage anxiety (Eubanks Higgins et al., 2013; see also Chapter 1, Appendix 1A).

Anxiety is "a combination of normal psychophysiological reactions, such as feelings of apprehension, tension, and nervousness in response to stressful situations that seem threatening or uncertain" (Kuo et al., 2016, p. 19). Some anxiety is necessary for peak performance, but too little or too much decreases performance. In the absence of sufficient anxiety, a person would lack the motivation to prepare adequately, but as anxiety increases past a person's capacity to cope, it becomes debilitating (e.g., lowered self-efficacy).

MacFarlane et al. (2016) found highly anxious genetic counseling students "were more likely to describe problematic supervisory relationships, appreciate the supervisor's ability to help them when they get stuck in sessions, and feel their anxiety had a negative effect on their performance in general and in supervision" (p. 742). High anxiety can cause students to shut down in supervision and genetic counseling sessions, become distracted by thoughts of how their supervisor or client is evaluating them, focus more on their supervisor's evaluation than on building counseling skills or getting the most they can from the rotation, feel overwhelmed during supervision meetings, and/or fail to clarify misunderstandings.

Types and Sources of Anxiety

Kuo et al. (2016) identified three major types of student anxiety:

Anticipatory—future-oriented anxiety from expectations that something bad will happen and the individual is helpless to predict, control, or achieve desired results.

Approval—desire for recognition, acceptance, and approval by supervisors, clients, and others, coupled with a belief that one will not receive that approval.

Dominance—reaction to authority and power. Supervision is a hierarchical power relationship in which supervisors control rewards and influence processes and outcomes. A key factor is whether the supervisor's influence is supportive or coercive.

Box 14.3 lists several potential sources of student anxiety in clinical supervision.

Behaviors Suggestive of Anxiety

Ultimately, effective supervision involves a process that encourages students to extend beyond their comfort zone and push through anxiety, without becoming overwhelmed (Kuo et al., 2016, p. 19).

BOX 14.3 Sources of Student Anxiety in Supervision

Receipt of feedback/evaluation (Kuo et al., 2016)

Unclear expectations (Kuo et al., 2016)

Supervisor anxiety (Kuo et al., 2016)

Performance anxiety (fears not meeting *internally* set performance standard) (Liddle, 1986)

Personal issues (e.g., difficulty with authority, unprocessed grief over a major loss) (Liddle, 1986)

Deficiencies in the supervision relationship (e.g., student does not feel safe, understood, and/or supported) (Liddle, 1986)

Fears *punishment* from clients and/or supervisor for mistakes (Liddle, 1986)

Competition with peers (Costa, 1994)

Resentment of taking on the learner role (Costa, 1994)

Challenge of learning different supervisor approaches (Costa, 1994)

Initial awkwardness in using genetic counseling techniques (Costa, 1994)

Supervisor games that include the following (McIntosh et al., 2006):

- "I won't tell you what to do but I will say you're doing it wrong"—supervisor intentionally provides ambiguous instructions, does not provide assistance, and criticizes the student for not doing the task "right."
- "Letters are due yesterday"—supervisor changes expectations (specifically deadlines) to exert power over the student.
- "Do it exactly as I do it"—supervisor requires student to do everything precisely as the supervisor does things to demonstrate control.

Sources: Costa, L. (1994). Reducing anxiety in live supervision. *Counselor Education and Supervision, 34*, 30–40; Kuo, H. J., Connor, A., Landon, T. J., & Chen, R. K. (2016). Managing anxiety in clinical supervision. *Journal of Rehabilitation, 82*, 18–27; Liddle, B. J. (1986). Resistance in supervision: A response to perceived threat. *Counselor Education and Supervision, 26*, 117–127; McIntosh, N., Dircks, A., Fitzpatrick, J., & Shuman, C. (2006). Games in clinical genetic counseling supervision. *Journal of Genetic Counseling, 15*, 225–244 (pp. 234–235).

Supervisors' awareness of their own and the student's emotional arousal is the first step in that process. Kuo et al. identify three general ways students manifest anxiety:

> *Moves away from*—The student escapes or hides (e.g., closed posture, does not maintain active listening, is late, stops responding to email, and misses deadlines).
>
> *Moves against*—The student constantly disagrees with the supervisor, argues, and criticizes.
>
> *Moves toward*—The student agrees with everything the supervisor says or suggests. This pattern can sometimes be difficult to notice because a certain amount of agreement is expected in a learning environment. Excessive and/or quick agreement, however, can be problematic if the student does not logically process what they are hearing and then becomes confused when they try to use the supervisor's suggestions. Agreement can also be problematic when a student becomes overly dependent on the supervisor's ideas.

McIntosh et al. (2006, pp. 231–232) identified student behaviors that may or may not be intentional and indicate ways they cope poorly with anxiety:

- "Poor me"—The student heavily criticizes their own work to gain more praise and reassurance from the supervisor.
- "Cozy intern"—An underperforming student tries to establish a peer relationship with the supervisor in hopes of preventing negative evaluations.
- "Controlling feedback"—The student begins debriefing sessions with a long self-assessment, which prevents the supervisor from having time to offer corrective feedback.
- "Challenge me"—The student asks questions about the supervisor's skills or knowledge to control the focus of supervision.

Anxiety Management Strategies

Several strategies may be beneficial for helping students manage their anxiety:

- Engage in ongoing assessment of the supervision relationship and initiate discussion of the relationship to gauge student anxiety and how the student is coping.
- Spend time building rapport to help normalize anxiety (MacFarlane et al., 2016; Wherley et al., 2015).
- Balance support and guidance to build a working alliance. "Secure supervisor–supervisee attachment has a protective effect on students who experience non-productive anxiety" (Kuo et al., 2016, p. 24).
- Discuss your expectations often. Clearly stated expectations will "place limits on what often seems like a 'limitless' environment" (Fall & Sutton, 2004, p. 74). Explain why your expectations matter. A supervision agreement will begin the discussion process.
- Feedback is a focal point for anxiety. Maintain a balance between reinforcing strengths and providing corrective feedback. Use an evocative approach to encourage student self-evaluation and to shape their self-feedback to be balanced and accurate (see Chapter 7).
- Encourage students to learn and use proactive approaches to manage anxiety, such as mindfulness and self-care strategies (MacFarlane et al., 2016; see also Chapter 12, this volume).
- Discuss/normalize psychotherapy as beneficial for managing debilitating anxiety (MacFarlane et al., 2016).
- In some cases, you may want to work with the student's genetic counseling program leadership to provide resources to help support the student.

Fall and Sutton (2004, pp. 74–75) recommend encouraging students to talk about their fears:

- Show that you understand how challenging their situation is and communicate affirmation and support.
- Work collaboratively and in a consultative style.
- Set clear goals to define specifically what is expected of them.
- Self-disclose your own feelings of anxiety during your training to normalize their situation.
- Consider using humor to alleviate anxiety. I find self-deprecating humor has a more positive effect. Avoid humor a student might perceive as making fun of them or a client.

Example of Addressing One Source of Student Anxiety: Multiple Supervisors

Genetic counseling fieldwork frequently involves multiple supervisors working with a single student, and this experience can raise student anxiety. Genetic counseling students have commented on the difficulty of integrating diverse and, at times, contradictory feedback, remembering and being responsive to each supervisor's expectations, and differentiating feedback based on stylistic differences from feedback about essential skills (Hendrickson et al., 2002; MacFarlane et al., 2016).

Individual Strategies

Several individual strategies may help you address student anxiety over having multiple supervisors:

- Explain the advantages of having multiple supervisors, including experiencing different styles of counseling, such as there is not a single "right" way to do genetic counseling, they will learn different perspectives, and they will receive a broader range of feedback (MacFarlane et al., 2016).

- Invite your student to express their concerns about having multiple supervisors. Help them anticipate potential challenges and discuss ways to address those challenges. Possible challenges include student anxiety and distress over supervisors who have contradictory expectations; trying to "cater" to supervisor preferences, but having difficulty remembering those preferences; receiving evaluations from supervisors who had such limited contact with the student that their evaluation may be inaccurate or incomplete; difficulty coordinating with multiple supervisors' schedules; and lack of communication among the various supervisors (MacFarlane et al., 2016). It is also possible that feedback across supervisors is inconsistent due to some of the factors previously discussed in this chapter, such as countertransference.
- Watch for student distress and anxiety, and intervene to help them manage their reactions.

Systemic Strategies

Certain procedural and logistical strategies may be helpful:

- Supervisors at a site could occasionally observe each other's genetic counseling to learn how they approach their work in similar and different ways. This activity would allow them to better understand what students are experiencing.
- Supervisors at a site could periodically meet during the rotation to discuss their impressions of the student's work and challenges due to having multiple supervisors.
- Appointing a "lead supervisor" would allow the student to call upon that individual for assistance in consolidating and integrating feedback from different supervisors.
- When possible, training programs and fieldwork sites should avoid having multiple supervisors in a first rotation because novice students are more likely to be overwhelmed by different expectations and discrepant feedback.

Closing Thoughts

With regard to supervision challenges, if you treat your students and yourself the way your treat clients, you will be more likely to have good outcomes, so

- be planful and strategic;
- encourage a collaborative process;
- recognize there are no "routine" students;
- customize your approach to each student; and
- celebrate your students' victories and your victories, however small.

Learning Activities

Most learning activities can be adapted for dyad or small group discussions or for written exercises. Time estimates are provided for discussions, but additional time should be allotted for large group processing.

Activity 14.1 Conflict in Supervision

Part I: Discussion

In small groups, describe a conflict you personally encountered or expect to encounter in supervision. Do not identify any involved parties other than yourself.

Next, identify strategies for addressing each conflict.

Estimated time: 30 minutes

Part II: Role Plays

Triads take turns as supervisor, student, and observer for three of the situations described in Part I. After each role play, the observer and student give feedback to the supervisor about how they addressed the issue.

Estimated time: 30 minutes

Activity 14.2 Countertransference Self-Reflection

With a partner:

- Describe one genetic counseling supervision issue, situation, or type of student that is/would be most likely to make you feel anxious, detached, annoyed, etc., or to engage in some sort of behavior that is not characteristic of you.
- Discuss what you think would make you react that way.
- Identify ways you might alter your perceptions to manage your reaction.

Estimated time: 20 minutes

Adapted from Weil, J. (2010). Countertransference: Making the unconscious conscious. In B. S. LeRoy, P. McCarthy Veach, & D. M. Bartels (Eds.), *Genetic counseling practice: Advanced concepts and skills* (pp. 175–200). Wiley-Blackwell.

Activity 14.3 Addressing Countertransference

Part I: Discussion

In small groups, for each scenario, imagine you are the supervisor. Discuss how you are feeling and what you would say/do.

Scenario: You are supervising a student in their third rotation. The student just does not quite want to do charting and client letters the way you have asked them to. The student shows you a draft of a chart note and letter and says, "You know, I don't write the way you want me to. The way I've written this, it really doesn't fit to put it in the format like you wanted." You're thinking, "What the heck is this? Can't you just follow simple instructions?"

Scenario: Your student wrote you an angry email 24 hours after you had provided some pointed corrective feedback. One of the comments in the email was, "Of course you had to say those things—you never liked me. I knew from the beginning that's how it was going to be. You never liked me." You can't believe the student completely missed the point of your feedback.

Scenario: You are supervising a student who continually has this look on their face when you answer questions. It's a laughing/frowning, questioning incredulity, and you interpret that look as the student thinking you are the stupidest genetic counselor on the planet.

Scenario: You have worked several days with your student. Although you haven't actually "crossed swords," the student has been a kind of perpetual low-grade irritant. The reason is, the student is pretty self-confident—a little too overconfident about their skills. You think if you'd had that attitude with your supervisors, they would have sent you home.

Estimated time: 30 minutes

Part II: Role Plays

Triads take turns as supervisor, student, and observer for the situations described in Part I. After each role play, the observer and student give feedback to the supervisor about how they addressed the issue.

Estimated time: 45 minutes

All scenarios are modified from Slater, R., McCarthy Veach, P., & Li, Z. (2012). Recognizing and managing countertransference in the college classroom: An exploration of expert teachers' experiences. *Innovative Higher Education, 38*, 3–17.

Activity 14.4 Student Anxiety

In dyads or small groups, discuss the following:

- What specific factors tend to raise student anxiety in your setting? (For student participants, talk about your most recent rotation setting.)
- What cues tell you a student is anxious?
- Which of *your* characteristics/behaviors might prompt student anxiety?
- What strategies have you found or do you think are effective for dealing with student anxiety?

Estimated time: 25 minutes

Activity 14.5 Addressing Student Anxiety

Part I: Discussion

In small groups, discuss how you would address each of the following scenarios:

Scenario: Your student is very anxious and makes factual mistakes in interpreting test results to clients. The more that you point out these mistakes and ask your student to correct them for the client, the more anxious and unsure the student becomes, and the more mistakes the student makes.

Scenario: You are supervising a student who never admits they do not know something even when it is obvious the student is in over their head.

Scenario: This is your third supervision meeting with your novice student. The student is telling you about their case prep in a very disorganized, unfocused manner. They talk nonstop, presenting a great amount of detail but no critical reflection.

Scenario: At mid-rotation, your student tells you they are feeling discouraged. They had spoken to a classmate whom you supervised last year. Their classmate was able to do more parts of the counseling sessions than they have been able to do so far.

Estimated time: 25 minutes

Part II: Role Plays

Take turns as supervisor, student, and observer for the situations described in Part I. After each role play, the observer and student give feedback to the supervisor about how they addressed the issue.

Estimated time: 30–45 minutes

15

Supervision Delivery Methods

KATIE WUSIK

Objectives

- Describe supervision delivery methods relevant to genetic counseling practice (live, self-report, remote, standardized patient, and peer supervision).
- Review advantages and challenges of each method.
- Demonstrate application of delivery methods to various genetic counseling supervision situations.

Genetic counselor supervisors first and foremost have a responsibility to ensure that students are prepared and demonstrate the skill to share genetic information (content) that is relevant, thorough, and accurate. Genetic counseling is primarily a medical profession and as such, experiences with clients are often short term and information-focused by necessity. During the early stages of training, live supervision of genetic counseling students by their clinical supervisors is required by the Accreditation Council for Genetic Counseling (ACGC), and genetic counseling graduate programs are instructed to ensure clients are not seen independently by students who have yet to demonstrate mastery of skills pertinent to the client interaction (ACGC, 2019a). It is therefore not surprising, based on these standards, that live supervision is the most common supervision method in genetic counseling (Lindh et al., 2003; Masunga et al., 2014). As discussed later, however, live supervision is not without its limitations (Hendrickson et al., 2002; Lindh et al., 2003; MacFarlane et al., 2016).

The ACGC also encourages supervisors to use a graduated supervision plan that allows students to develop autonomy in preparation for professional practice (ACGC, 2019a; Wherley et al., 2015). Genetic counselor supervisor competencies include using "supervisory methods appropriate to [a] student's level of conceptual development, training and experience" (Eubanks Higgins et al., 2013, p. 55).

Most genetic counseling clinical supervisors will utilize multiple supervision delivery methods to achieve students' successful transition to practicing professionals (Grove et al., 2019; Hendrickson et al., 2002; L. Kessler et al., 2021; Lindh et al., 2003; MacFarlane et al., 2016; Masunga et al., 2014). In addition, due to setting, specialty, and/or availability of supervisors, it may not be possible to utilize live supervision in which the supervisor is in the room with the student as the predominant modality in all cases (e.g., telemedicine, supervisor and student in different locations, nonclinical rotations, etc.). This chapter focuses on supervision delivery methods relevant to genetic counseling supervision with an emphasis on their practical implementation in various settings.

Live Supervision

In genetic counseling, the term *live supervision* typically refers to a supervisor being present in the room with the student and client (Hendrickson et al., 2002; Lindh et al., 2003; Masunga et al., 2014). Different variations of live supervision include the supervisor present for the entire session or a portion of the session (Lindh et al., 2003), the supervisor and student co-counsel the client, and the supervisor remains silent throughout the interaction (Masunga et al., 2014). Observing remotely through a one-way mirror has also been documented (Hendrickson et al., 2002; Masunga et al., 2014), but it is used much less frequently (Masunga et al., 2014).

Live Supervision Advantages

One advantage of live supervision is it can be adapted to provide varying degrees of autonomy for a student. Genetic counselor supervisors have reported using different combinations of techniques depending on the student's developmental level (Lindh et al., 2003; Masunga et al., 2014). For example, an intermediate student may have achieved the ability to independently obtain a pedigree and medical intake but still be working to master psychosocial counseling skills. The student could complete the pedigree and intake autonomously, with the supervisor joining the session later to provide co-counseling about, for instance, the decision to proceed with testing. Alternatively, the supervisor could be present the entire session but remain silent, only intervening if the student requests or needs assistance (Hendrickson et al., 2002; MacFarlane et al., 2016; Smith, 2009). For a more advanced student nearing graduation, the supervisor may have little or no need to intervene in the session. In that situation, to ensure client safety and promote student independence, observation through a one-way mirror may be ideal (Smith, 2009).

Another advantage of the more common variations of live supervision is they provide an immediate safety net for the student, who can invite supervisory assistance during the client interaction (Hendrickson et al., 2002; MacFarlane et al., 2016). An advantage specific to co-counseling is that it allows the student to participate by performing skills they have mastered and also observe the supervisor modeling more complex skills within the same interaction (Smith, 2009). In addition, students can attempt small pieces of a more complex skill, gradually building competence and confidence, until they are able to perform the skill in its entirety (Borders et al., 2006). For example, a novice student may be anxious about completing an entire medical intake in a new specialty. Together, the supervisor and the student could break the intake into smaller sections. The student starts with one small section and takes on additional sections in subsequent sessions until they are completing the entire medical intake for every client. Other skills, such as obtaining family history and constructing the pedigree, can also be broken into more manageable, successive steps: The student listens as the supervisor obtains family history information, and then the student draws their own pedigree for later comparison; the student draws the basic structure of the family tree, but the supervisor asks targeted medical history questions relevant to the encounter; and the student obtains the complete family history and constructs a pedigree. Note that supervisors may also benefit from live supervision because this delivery mode encourages the supervisor to practice self-reflection (Hendrickson et al., 2002).

Live Supervision Challenges

Live supervision within a genetic counseling session may present logistical challenges such as lack of facility resources (e.g., one-way mirror for observation) or supervisor time. Live supervision often requires the supervisor to provide guidance about case preparation, attend the session, and conduct a debriefing following a client interaction (Hendrickson et al., 2002). These activities can be time-intensive (Hendrickson et al., 2002; Lindh et al., 2003; Masunga et al., 2014). If the supervisor's time is limited and they are supervising two students, they could consider triadic supervision (Berg et al., 2018). In triadic supervision, a supervisor would provide live supervision within genetic counseling sessions individually but meet with both students together to conduct case preparations and debriefings. This strategy is more time-efficient and has an added benefit that students participate in feedback and guidance processes on both of their cases (Lewis, Erby, et al., 2017).

Live supervision can raise student anxiety (Hendrickson et al., 2002; Lindh et al., 2003; MacFarlane et al., 2016). Excessive anxiety may diminish student performance and lead to dependency (e.g., shaping their genetic counseling to conform to their supervisor's style) (Hendrickson et al., 2002; MacFarlane et al., 2016). Some students report deferring to the supervisor or relying too frequently on the supervisor's ability to answer patient questions (Hendrickson et al., 2002; MacFarlane et al., 2016). Importantly, supervisors must determine if a student's behavior is a pattern or specific to a particular scenario. For example, it could be expected that a student would defer to their supervisor for more complex aspects of a counseling session early in a rotation and/or in a new area of specialty practice. However, if a student is still exhibiting this behavior after several weeks in the rotation, this suggests a pattern that may impact the ability to achieve supervision outcomes such as independence and formulation of a personal style (Anderson et al., 1995; Bubenzer & West, 1993; Wherley et al., 2015). Strategies to address student anxiety are discussed in Chapter 14.

During live supervision, supervisors may become too involved in client interactions; have difficulty determining when to intervene; intervene too much; or, after intervening, be unable to pass the interaction back to the student (Hendrickson et al., 2002; Macfarlane et al., 2016). At the beginning of the supervision relationship, students and supervisors should work together to establish ways in which the student feels comfortable signaling the need for supervisor intervention during a session (see Chapter 7). For example, a student may make eye contact with the supervisor or may simply tell the client that the supervisor will discuss a specific question in more detail. These strategies allow students some control in the supervisory relationship. If intervention is needed, a supervisor should redirect the session back to the student as soon as possible by prompting the student to answer the next question (Hendrickson et al., 2002) or directing the student where to pick up the conversation. If a supervisor is hesitant to return the reins of the session to the student because of uncertainty about their knowledge, the supervisor should consider having the student prepare an outline prior to the next client interaction (Hendrickson et al., 2002). Last, to promote the student's interactions with the client, it is helpful for the supervisor to be positioned so they are not in the client's direct line of site or for the student to be positioned closer to the client (Hendrickson et al., 2002).

Other Considerations Regarding Live Supervision

Additional challenges that may need the supervisor's attention include the impact of involvement of multiple practicing professionals on the client's reaction to the student. Students have noted their roles decrease when a physician is present (Hendrickson et al., 2002), and this may extend to other professionals as well. Supervisors should consider how and when to protect the student's autonomy and support their role in the clinic. To help prevent a negative reaction from clients to student involvement, supervisors could consider adding a description of student participation in pre-clinic information, address the importance of student learning, and/or highlight the student's knowledge and training to date (Hendrickson et al., 2002).

Self-Report

Self-report refers to a student interacting with a client alone, followed by reporting various aspects of the interaction and the student's own reflections to the supervisor (Smith, 2009). Self-report appears to be a growing method of supervision in genetic counseling. In 2003, 9.3% of supervisors reported using the method with beginning students, and 38.9% reported using it with advanced students (Lindh et al., 2003); in 2014, supervisors reported higher utilization with both beginning (46.6%) and advanced (61.2%) students, although it was unclear if supervisors were using self-report exclusively or paired with some amount of live supervision (Masunga et al., 2014).

Self-Report Advantages

Two of the supervision outcomes identified in the Reciprocal-Engagement Model of Supervision (see Chapter 1) are students apply information independently and students engage in self-reflective practice (Wherley et al., 2015). Self-report can be an effective method for promoting these outcomes. Self-report may also have the advantage of being less time-intensive for supervisors because they do not have to be present at entire sessions for every client.

Self-Report Challenges

The most commonly noted barriers to using self-report include genetic counseling supervisors' concerns about client safety, the amount of time needed for debriefing following the session, and concerns that the method is not effective for training students (Masunga et al., 2014). Relatedly, some institutions or rotation sites may have policies limiting the situations in which a student is allowed to provide genetic counseling services by themself.

Studies of self-report in mental health counseling have found additional potential challenges, including concerns with supervisees withholding information from their supervisors (Ladany et al., 1996; Mehr et al., 2010). Supervisee nondisclosure may be more likely in the absence of a strong supervisor–supervisee relationship. Supervisees may feel more comfortable expressing mistakes or concerns when they have a positive relationship with their supervisor (Mehr et al., 2010). The relationship between the supervisor and the student is a key component of genetic counseling supervision (Wherley et al., 2015; see Chapter 1), and genetic counseling student self-efficacy has been positively associated with the student's rating of the relationship with their current supervisor (Caldwell et al., 2018b). Therefore, the supervisor–student relationship may be especially important when utilizing self-report.

The student's developmental level may also affect their ability to engage in the supervision process (Pearson, 2001; see also Chapter 5, this volume). Novices may have more difficulty determining what to share and what types of feedback to request (Knox, 2015) compared to advanced students (Loganbill et al., 1982; Stoltenberg & McNeill, 2011).

Integrating Self-Report into Genetic Counseling Supervision

Within the boundaries of clinic policy and with a focus on client safety, self-report can be an important supervision technique to ensure a gradual transition from student to practitioner. Self-report may be best utilized with more advanced students, for specific genetic counseling skills, or in combination with live supervision during which the supervisor is silent. Supervisors might consider using a self-report approach for a defined portion of the genetic counseling session and increase its use as the student's skills advance. This approach corresponds to the ACGC's (2019a) recommendations to utilize a graduated supervision plan.

Additional self-report strategies include asking students to self-reflect and summarize their thoughts prior to discussing a client interaction during supervision (Pearson, 2001, Students & Pearson, 2004; see also Chapter 9, this volume). Supervisors can provide guidance during supervision meetings with respect to what information should be shared. Supervisors might also consider using audio or video recording in conjunction with self-report. Recordings are not widely used in genetic counseling due to barriers such as lack of equipment, concerns about clients' reactions, and logistical issues such as client consent (Masunga et al., 2014). Recordings, when feasible, can help supervisors determine if a student's self-assessments are accurate and eliminate concerns about their withholding information; however, listening to recordings can be time-consuming. Supervisors might consider having only the student review their recordings, or supervisors could review small sections of the recorded sessions to decease the time burden.

Standardized Patients

Generally, a standardized patient (also known as a simulated patient) is an individual who is trained to take on the role of a patient/

client (Lewis, Bohnert, et al., 2017). The person could be portraying their own prior experiences, or they could be acting from a scripted role (Barrows, 1993). Standardized patients provide a relatively consistent scenario each time, even when variables such as the student differ (Barrows, 1993).

Standardized Patient Advantages

Multiple human services fields use standardized patients (Barrows, 1993; Betcher, 2010; Hayden et al., 2014; Meghani & Ferm, 2021; Paramasivan & Khoo, 2019; Ruiz-Moral et al., 2017), including genetic counseling (Andoni et al., 2018; Erby et al., 2011; R. Holt et al., 2013; Kessler et al., 2021; Redlinger-Grosse et al., 2021). Some studies have shown higher quality interactions with clients, greater retention of training (Betcher, 2010), and improved ability to show empathy and talk about client emotions (Selman et al., 2017). In one study of nursing students, however, no differences in mastery of clinical skills were found between groups that had variable percentages of standardized patients, when accounting for clinical training experience (Hayden et al., 2014). Genetic counseling students have reported that standardized patients are helpful in building skills (Holt et al., 2013).

Standardized patient experiences may be more structured than typical role plays to facilitate more uniform assessment of students (Barrows, 1993; International Nursing Association for Clinical Simulation and Learning Standards Committee, 2016; Lewis, Bohnert, et al., 2017). The Association of Standardized Patient Educators created a best practice document that provides guidance for standardized patient encounters (Lewis, Bohnert, et al., 2017). Training for role portrayal should include explanation of objectives and practice of the scenario followed by targeted feedback (Lewis, Bohnert, et al., 2017).

In genetic counseling, most graduate programs surveyed reported utilizing standardized patients (Kessler et al., 2021). Some authors propose using them to help students develop basic skills, with students moving on to real clients once they have mastered those skills (Roche & Greb, 2016). Current genetic counseling program accreditation standards allow a small percentage of a student's required participatory cases to involve standardized patients (ACGC, 2019a). One advantage of this method is that it ensures all students experience certain situations that cannot be guaranteed to occur during rotations. For example, standardized patient scenarios could involve a positive genetic test results disclosure (Kessler et al., 2021), giving unexpected news (Andoni et al., 2018), pre-test counseling, and negative genetic testing results disclosure (Kessler et al., 2021). The ACGC (n.d.) notes that supervisors may serve as standardized patients if they receive training and if outcomes are created for the encounter.

Integrating Standardized Patients into Genetic Counseling Supervision

Individually or in a group at their site, supervisors could develop standardized scenarios specific to the rotation learning objectives and use standardized patients in a variety of ways during the rotation. For example, supervisors might use a standardized patient at the beginning for an advanced student. If the student meets every objective for the scenario, they may be able to progress toward using self-report more quickly. The standardized patient experience may allow supervisors to feel more confident that the student is prepared to meet client needs. On the other hand, if the student does not meet all the objectives, a supervisor may wish to use a more gradual transition from live supervision variations to self-report.

In genetic counseling training, the use of standardized patients in nonclinical fieldwork may also be beneficial. Consider, for example, supervisors working in a laboratory who explain abnormal microarray results to health care providers. They could utilize standardized patients to ensure students are able to accurately call out the results and respond to common questions (accuracy, validity, recommended follow-up, etc.) prior to allowing them to call out results independently.

Peer Group Supervision

Peer Groups for Professionals

Peer group supervision in genetic counseling generally refers to a set of professionals who meet regularly to provide each other mentorship (Kennedy, 2000a). The supervision may be leader-led by an experienced genetic counselor or a professional with a different training background, such as psychology, social work, or marriage/family therapy (Kennedy, 2000b; Townend, 2005; Zahm et al., 2008). Potential benefits of peer group supervision include improved self-awareness and ability to engage in self-reflective practice, advancement of psychosocial counseling skills, management of emotions related to work with clients and with student supervisees, navigation of ethical dilemmas, and continued development of personal style (Bernhardt et al., 2010; Miranda et al., 2016; Resta, 2002; Zahm et al., 2008).

Researchers have suggested genetic counselor supervisors consider formation of peer supervision groups that focus, at least in part, on supervision skills and issues (Siskind & Atzinger, 2019; Wherley et al., 2015). These groups could easily span both client-facing and non-client-facing specialties to consider the skills used by all supervisors.

Considerations for developing a peer supervision group include determination of whether to have a leader, the group structure, and how the group will be governed. For example, who will comprise the group, and will the group be open to new members? Several reports of peer group supervision in genetic counseling mention that groups vary in size, ranging from six genetic counselors to no size restrictions (Kennedy, 2000b; Middleton et al., 2007; Zahm et al., 2008). Group members may have similar or a mixture of experience levels (Kennedy, 2000b). Other considerations in formation of a peer supervision group include whether there should be attendance requirements, length and frequency of meetings, and whether there are any costs to members or their employers for participation (Kennedy, 2000a; Middleton et al., 2007; Zahm et al., 2008). Descriptions of peer supervision groups typically mention creation of a safe space (Bosco, 2000; Hiller & Rosenfield, 2000) or trust within the group (Kennedy, 2000a; Lewis, Erby, et al., 2017).

Peer Groups for Students

A graduate program or fieldwork site may also consider incorporating peer groups into genetic counseling student training and supervision. Programs may utilize peer supervision with student cohorts to promote group debriefing and self-reflective practice. Examples of activities include a check-in during which students briefly share how things are going in their rotations and whether they would like some group time to discuss a specific issue; informal and formal presentations of client cases; and role-playing of challenging situations.

In a site at which several students rotate at the same time, supervisors could use peer group supervision. When creating a student peer supervision group, it is important to consider how to build trust among the participants, logistics such as confidentiality, and ways of managing group dynamics. When students are rotating for only a few weeks at a site, peer supervision may not be the most appropriate method, depending on the students' relationships with one another.

Peer Observation and Feedback

Peer observation and feedback has been used for differing purposes with practicing genetic counselors (e.g., improved self-awareness and completion of critical elements of a session) (Goldsmith et al., 2011; Secton et al., 2013). Peer observation and feedback may complement other supervision delivery methods for students. For smaller groups of students, or in instances in which peer group supervision may not be feasible, variations such as vertical supervision or paired peer supervision (Berninger et al., 2020; Lindh et al., 2003) could be considered. In the most basic form of vertical supervision, an advanced student would receive training from the supervisor on supervision skills and, in turn, provide supervision to a novice student (Curtis et al., 2016; Minnes, 1989). In paired peer supervision, students would be grouped in dyads to provide feedback to each other (Berninger et al., 2020). Paired students may have similar or different levels of experience and would also have an individual relationship with a supervisor (Berninger et al., 2020). Paired peer supervision is like the triadic supervision method described previously in this chapter; however, in paired peer supervision, students have a greater responsibility for providing feedback to each other because they would observe their partner's sessions.

Although students have reported decreased anxiety when another student provides supervision and feedback (Dickerson et al., 2017; Sevenhuysen et al., 2014, 2015; Tai et al., 2016), concerns with supervisees not receiving expert feedback and client safety have been raised (Sevenhuysen et al., 2014). An adaptation of these methods for genetic counseling peer supervision is to have a supervisor present during supervision meetings to provide support and guidance around student interactions and feedback or have the student reflect on their peer's feedback prior to a meeting with the supervisor.

Remote Supervision

Genetic counselors who have not served as supervisors have noted distance from a graduate program as a barrier to providing supervision (Berg et al., 2018). Remote supervision methods may help alleviate this barrier. Many of the supervision delivery methods discussed thus far are also applicable for remote supervision. For example, live remote supervision may refer to a supervisor monitoring a client interaction from a different location (telephone or video feed). Live remote supervision was utilized by less than 5% of supervisors in a study conducted in 2014, with the most common barrier being lack of suitable facilities (Masunga et al., 2014). Noteworthy, however, is that almost twice the number of supervisors were interested in using remote live supervision if barriers did not exist (Masunga et al., 2014). As the use of telemedicine and other remote service delivery models continues to increase, remote live supervision may become a more prevalent modality.

Peer supervision, standardized patients, and self-report could all be implemented remotely. Non-client-facing rotations could be easily adapted to remote supervision, too. Entirely remote industry lab rotations have been described in genetic counseling (Grove et al., 2019). Unknown, however, is the extent to which supervision quality and content may be impacted as interactions increasingly take place remotely.

When providing remote supervision, supervisors should take care to emphasize relationship building and communication (Martin et al., 2017). When feasible, the first supervision meeting should be conducted in person (Martin et al., 2017). If that is not possible, videoconferencing may be a viable alternative (Martin et al., 2017). Both supervisors and students should receive training on the platform that will be involved (Sahebi, 2020; Schultz et al., 2021). Supervisors and students should discuss how to troubleshoot technical problems that may occur during supervision meetings and/or client interactions (Martin et al., 2017). Supervisors should also consider how they will be involved during remote client interactions (Schultz et al., 2021). For example, a supervisor may remain silent by turning off their audio. On a videoconference, they may also turn off their video to help the student build rapport and acknowledge the student's authority.

Body language may be less obvious on video and absent in telecommunication. It may be difficult to determine to whom the client is directing a question, increasing student anxiety about who should field the question. Typical supervision signals involving body language (e.g., student looks at supervisor for help) are also difficult to use. Supervisors may need to provide students with alternate suggestions for how to ask for help.

Example

Sasha is calling Dr. Patel, a primary care provider, with microarray results that identified a pathogenic deletion for one of Dr. Patel's pediatric patients. At the beginning of the call, Sasha introduced herself and noted that Mikel, her supervisor, was also present. During their pre-call discussion, Sasha and Mikel agreed that Mikel would join the call muted. Mikel felt comfortable with Sasha's plan for discussing the implications of the deletion. However, they agreed if Sasha needed any help during the call, she could ask Mikel directly to answer specific questions. As the call begins, Dr. Patel has many technical questions about the ability of the microarray to detect the specific deletion breakpoints. Sasha recognizes she is not able to answer Dr. Patel's questions and says, "Dr. Patel, I am going to ask Mikel to address your questions regarding the breakpoints." At the mention of his name, Mikel provides additional details before turning the call back over to Sasha to wrap up the discussion. After the call, Sasha mentions that she felt relieved they had a plan for how she could ask Mikel for help.

Remote supervision may also refer to emerging areas of study, such as the use of email as a supervisory delivery method (Luke & Gordon, 2016). Email communication may be used for client-facing rotations (remote or in-person) in advance of or following client interactions to discuss case preparation or to determine follow-up activities after an appointment. Email may also be used extensively in remote non-client-facing rotations. For example, students completing a laboratory rotation may review incoming test orders for appropriateness. After reviewing a test order, they may email their supervisor with their case analysis, with the supervisor providing written feedback. The types of supervision delivery methods used within remote rotations in genetic counseling have not yet been described (Grove et al., 2019).

Although email may be commonly used for supervision interactions in the genetic counseling field, caution is necessary because tone and intent are difficult to interpret in written communication. In addition, confidentiality regarding the client and the student *must* be safeguarded (e.g., emails may be forwarded to other parties who are not the intended recipient). Supervisors should discuss appropriate use of email with the student and check with their institution about policies regarding sending secure/encrypted emails outside of their institution. Emailing protected health information outside one's institution without appropriately implementing security measures may result in a Health Insurance Portability and Accountability Act violation, potentially incurring fines.

In the school counseling literature, limited research has been conducted to identify techniques supervisors employed when communicating via email (Gordon & Luke, 2012, 2013; Luke & Gordon, 2011). Suggested techniques include use of indirect statements (e.g., "Have you considered doing further research . . ." versus "Do this research now"), use of collective pronouns (e.g., we) to build the supervision working alliance, use of shared language with the supervisee, and modeling appropriate language (Luke & Gordon, 2016).

As with any type of supervision delivery method, remote supervision would ideally be complemented with a variety of methods, tailored to students' unique needs and goals. As technology and telemedicine advance, and supervisors and students become more familiar with logistics, it is reasonable to expect that remote supervision will become more common.

Closing Thoughts

All supervision delivery methods have advantages and challenges. Utilizing a mixture of supervision delivery methods, such as live supervision, self-report, peer supervision, standardized patients, and remote supervision, can help mitigate the challenges of any one method. Supervisors should work with each student to determine a suitable mix of delivery methods that will promote their development while also appropriately balancing the supervisor's needs, availability, and resources. The exact proportions of methods will vary across supervisors and specialties. Exposing students to a variety of delivery methods throughout their training has an added benefit of helping them become more versatile supervisors. Although most research on genetic counseling supervision delivery methods to date has focused on client-facing activities, many methods are broadly applicable to any type of genetic counseling interaction. Supervisors should strive to become comfortable with multiple delivery methods and view the array of available methods as tools to customize and personalize the experience for each student.

Learning Activities

Most learning activities can be adapted for dyad or small group discussions or for written exercises. Time estimates are provided for discussions, but additional time should be allotted for large group processing.

Activity 15.1 Reflections on Supervision Delivery Methods

With a partner or in small groups, discuss the following questions:

- Which supervision delivery method do you feel most comfortable with/are most likely to use?
- What are some of the reasons you feel this way?
- What are some challenges, and how might you overcome those challenges?

- Which supervision delivery method do you feel least comfortable with/least willing to use?
  - What are some of the reasons you feel this way?
  - What are some ways to become more comfortable?
- Which supervision delivery method presents the most barriers for you?
  - How could you overcome those barriers?

Estimated time: 20 minutes

Activity 15.2 Challenges in Live Supervision

With a partner or in small groups, discuss each of the following challenges to live supervision. Consider the extent to which you have had/are likely to have difficulties with each challenge, and brainstorm possible solutions for each one.

- Determining when to intervene in a case
- Intervening too often in a case
- Unable to pass the session back to the student

Estimated time: 20 minutes

Note: Dyad or small group participants could also role play discussing these challenges with a "student."

Activity 15.3 Client Reactions to Student Involvement

Part I: Discussion

In small specialty groups, create a description of student involvement for inclusion in pre-clinic information. Address how and when students may interact with clients, the purpose/importance of student learning, and students' training and supervision.

Estimated time: 20 minutes

Part II: Role Plays

Take turns as supervisor, student, client, and observers for role-play scenarios in which a client is resistant to student involvement. Each role play could emphasize a different reason for the client's resistance. Use information generated in Part I as a resource, as applicable to your practice setting. After each role play, the observers, client, and student give feedback to the supervisor about how they addressed the issue.

Estimated time: 30 minutes

Activity 15.4 Generating Questions for Self-Report

In dyads or small groups of supervisors practicing in similar specialties, generate questions to ask students when utilizing self-report methods. Consider generating questions that are specific to different sections of the client interaction, including, but not limited to, the following:

* Contracting
* Medical and family history
* Presentation of testing options
* Results disclosure

Estimated time: 30 minutes

Activity 15.5 Creating Guidelines for Peer Supervision Groups

In dyads or small groups, generate guidelines for implementation of a peer supervision group for students at your rotation site, institution, or graduate program. Include the following:

* Goals of the supervision
* Style of group (leader-led versus no leader)
* How to determine/generate meeting content

- Rules for attendance
- Frequency and length of meetings
- Norms regarding confidentiality, handling disagreements/ conflict, etc.

Estimated time: 30 minutes

Note: This activity can be used to create guidelines for a peer supervision group for supervisors.

Appendix

Instructional Tips for Building Supervision Training Opportunities

The following tips reflect general instructional approaches I have found effective for conducting workshops and classes on genetic counseling supervision.

Preparation

Structure

- Begin your presentation with an "advance organizer"—that is, what you intend to cover and how you intend to cover it. Advance organizers help orient the audience and move things along.
- Include a statement of participant learning objectives: "By the end of the class/presentation, participants will be able to . . . ."
- Pose your content as building tools to reflect upon and expand their supervision repertoire.
- An active approach enhances learning and retention. Keep lectures brief, and intersperse them with evocative questions and experiential activities.

- Evocative strategies yield rich thinking and discussion about topics. One strategy is to ask participants to share their ideas about a topic and then provide a mini lecture to reinforce and expand upon their thoughts.
- Begin with low-risk/less intimate disclosure topics before moving to higher risk/more intimate ones (e.g., asking participants to define *supervision* is a more cerebral activity than asking them to disclose conflicts they have experienced in supervision relationships).
- I recommend creating a presenter agenda that lists topics/ activities and estimated time for each. An agenda will help you determine how to situate various topics and activities. I encourage you, however, to be fluid enough to address topics as they arise from participants' questions and comments and to alter time allotments rather than sticking rigidly to a "script."
- Invite participants to choose their own partner for more intimate dyadic conversations.
- For group activities, mix up participants to encourage more interaction and thought sharing.
- Consider whether to put supervisors together for activities based on practice specialty. If you do so, point out what is similar and unique among the specialties during debriefing.
- Generally, I do not recommend dividing people into groups based on experience level. I believe everyone, regardless of their experience level, brings something to the table.
- I advise against presentations that mix supervisors and students. Even if the focus is solely on administrative issues (program expectations, evaluation forms, due process, etc.), full and honest participation may be stifled. There is also greater potential for an inadvertent breach of confidentiality.

Content

- Avoid overloading a presentation with too many topics because this will result in shallow consideration of important issues

and possibly hinder interaction if you and the participants feel rushed. "Less is more."
- Predetermine which sections of the presentation you will cut if you are running behind time.
- *Critical incidents* is an effective technique for creating scenarios based on participants' own experiences. Individual participants are instructed to write three or four sentences describing a supervision situation they have had or anticipate having. Collect their incidents and then distribute some to dyads or small groups for discussion.
- At the beginning of the class or workshop, create a list of participants' questions on a flip chart. Then try to address them throughout the presentation. If you invite participants' questions after first stating the objectives for the presentation, their questions will tend to be related to topics you plan to cover. Invite participants to add questions to the list during breaks in the class/workshop. As a closing activity, ask participants what their "answers" are to each question, and add your own ideas.
- A certain amount of repetition is good because it can deepen learning. I typically carry major themes (e.g., reflective practice) across topics and activities. This type of repetition also helps tie together seemingly disparate content.
- Specific examples help illustrate content.
- Practice (through experiential activities) concretizes concepts and skills and demonstrates where participants may be confused and/or challenged.

Presentation

Anonymity

- State and occasionally remind participants that genetic counseling is a relatively small community, so they should be careful when giving examples to not identify another supervisor or student. Remind individuals that some of their experiences may involve individuals who are in attendance (e.g., former students who are now supervisors).

Sensitivity

- People would rather talk than do, and usually they are anxious about being observed. Be encouraging of activities such as role playing. Anticipate some "groans." You may need to "nudge" participants to action.
- Provide reinforcement and encouragement/normalization when participants ask questions and make comments (e.g., "That's an excellent question that brings to light . . ."; "What you're describing is something supervisors at all levels of experience struggle with").
- Avoid asking anyone to "speak for" others from a cultural group (e.g., "Tom, what do male students think?").
- Limited self-disclosure of your own supervision experiences can help illustrate certain topics or skills and build rapport with your audience.
- Humor makes presentations more engaging, but be sure your humor is at yourself or an innocuous entity and not at a participant's expense.

Debriefing

- When conducting group discussions, invite volunteers to share their responses about more sensitive issues rather than asking everyone to share.
- Think about patterns/commonalities that emerge from participants' responses and verbally summarize those patterns.
- Try to call on as many different participants as possible— watch for individuals whose nonverbals suggest they may be interested in responding.

- Use an evocative approach to draw out participants' ideas when someone raises a question rather than answering all of the questions yourself. Summarize and refine the most pertinent ideas, and then add your own perspective.
- If challenged by a participant (e.g., "That strategy would take too much time"), ask the group, "What do you think about that? What are some ways to reduce the time it takes?"
- Some supervision content can be controversial (e.g., how much scaffolding to provide for students). Furthermore, stylistic differences will make some strategies more or less acceptable to different individuals. There is more than one way to "climb the mountain," so anticipate and acknowledge different perspectives.

Follow-Up

- Small group activities often yield important insights (e.g., feedback strategies that have been particularly effective). I suggest you ask each group to appoint a recorder of the discussion. Collect their notes, collate them, and share them with participants after the presentation. An option is to group the ideas by overarching themes before distributing them to participants.
- As a final activity, ask participants to spend 1 minute writing take-away messages for themselves. For example, "Two things I will do differently because of this workshop/class are . . . ."

References

Aamodt, P., Wetherill, L., Delk, P., Torres-Martinez, W., Vance, G. H., & Wesson, M. (2020). Positive and negative professionalism experiences of genetic counseling students in the United States and Canada. *Journal of Genetic Counseling, 30*, 478–492.

Accreditation Council for Genetic Counseling. (n.d.). *Guidance for COVID-19 related changes.* https://www.gceducation.org/guidance-for-covid-19-related-changes

Accreditation Council for Genetic Counseling. (2019a). *Practice-based competencies for genetic counselors.* https://www.gceducation.org/wp-content/uploads/2019/06/ACGC-Core-Competencies-Brochure_15_Web_REV-6-2019.pdf

Accreditation Council for Genetic Counseling. (2019b). *Standards of accreditation for graduate programs in genetic counseling.* https://www.gceducation.org/wp-content/uploads/2020/06/Revised-Standards-of-Accreditation_Final_Effective-10.1.19__6.17.20-Comp-Date-Rev-5.1-to-6.15.pdf

Acker, G. A. (2018). Self-care practices among social workers: Do they predict job satisfaction and turnover intention? *Social Work in Mental Health, 16*, 713–727.

Alonso, A. (1983). A developmental theory of psychodynamic supervision. *Clinical Supervisor, 1*, 23–26.

American Board of Genetic Counseling. (2004). *Requirements for graduate programs in genetic counseling seeking accreditation by the American Board of Genetic Counseling.*

American Psychological Association. (2014). *APA guidelines for clinical supervision in health service psychology.* http://apa.org/about/policy/guidelines-supervision.pdf

Ancis, J., & Ladany, N. (2010). A multicultural framework for counselor supervision: Knowledge and skills. In N. Ladany & L. Bradley (Eds.), *Counselor supervision* (4th ed., pp. 53–95). Routledge.

Anderson, L. M., Scrimshaw, S. C., Fullilove, M. T., Fielding, J. E., Normand, J., & the Task Force on Community Preventative Services. (2003). Culturally competent healthcare systems: A systematic review. *American Journal of Preventative Medicine, 24,* 68–79.

Anderson, S. A., Rigazio-DiGilio, S. A., & Kunkler, K. P. (1995). Training and supervision in family therapy: Current issues and future directions. *Family Relations, 44,* 489–500.

Andoni, L., Hobson, W. L., Carey, J. C., & Dent, K. M. (2018). Training methods for delivering difficult news in genetic counseling and genetics residency training programs. *Journal of Genetic Counseling, 27,* 1497–1505.

AnQuotes. (n.d.). *112 of most encouraging self-care quotes.* Retrieved April 12, 2021, from www.anquotes.com/self-care-quotes

Atzinger, C. L., Lewis, K., Martin, L. J., Yager, G., Ramstetter, C., & Wusik, K. (2014). The impact of supervision training on genetic counselor supervisory identity development. *Journal of Genetic Counseling, 23,* 1056–1065.

Australian Institute of Professional Counsellors. (2019, April 24). *Expectations and goals in clinical supervision.* Retrieved February 5, 2021, from https://www.counsellingconnection.com/index.php/2019/04/24/expectations-needs-and-goals-in-clinical-supervision

Baker, K. E. (2003). *Caring for ourselves.* American Psychological Association.

Bandura, A. (1982). Self-efficacy mechanism in human agency. *American Psychologist, 37,* 122–147.

Bannink, F. (2006). *Solution-focused interviewing.* Norton.

Barnett, J. E., & Molzon, C. H. (2014). Clinical supervision of psychotherapy: Essential ethics issues for supervisors and supervisees. *Journal of Clinical Psychology, 70,* 1051–1061.

Barrows, H. S. (1993). An overview of the uses of standardized patients for teaching and evaluating clinical skills. *Academic Medicine, 68,* 443–451.

Beagan, B. L. (2018). A critique of cultural competence: Assumptions, limitations, and alternatives. In C. Frisby & W. O'Donohue (Eds.), *Cultural competence in applied psychology* (pp. 123–138). Springer. https://doi.org/10.1007/978-3-319-78997-2_6

Behavioral Health Providers Association of New Mexico. (n.d.). *Models of clinical supervision, defined.* Retrieved January 23, 2021, from https://www.nmbhpa.org/clinical-supervision-implementation-guide/models-of-clinical-supervision-defined

Berg, J., Hoskovick, J., Shahrukh Hashmi, S., McCarthy Veach, P., Ownby, A., & Singletary, C. N. (2018). Relieving the bottleneck: An investigation of barriers to expansion of supervision networks at genetic counseling training programs. *Journal of Genetic Counseling, 27,* 241–251.

Bernard, J. M. (1979). Supervisor training: A discrimination model. *Counselor Education & Supervision, 19,* 60–68.

Bernard, J. M. (1997). The discrimination model. In C. E. Watkins (Ed.), *Handbook of psychotherapy supervision* (pp. 310–327). Wiley.

Bernard, J. M. (2010). Special issue on supervision: A reflection. *Canadian Journal of Counselling, 44,* 238–245.

Bernard, J. M., & Goodyear, R. K. (2014). *Fundamentals of clinical supervision* (5th ed.). Pearson.

Bernhardt, B. A., Silver, R., Rushton, C. H., Micco, E., & Geller, G. (2010). What keeps you up at night? Genetic professionals' distressing experiences in patient care. *Genetics in Medicine, 12,* 289–297.

Berninger, T., Nusbaum, R., Redlinger-Grosse, K., Davis, C., & Reiser, C. (2020). A narrative literature review: Growing the workforce through increased fieldwork capacity in genetic counseling training programs. *Journal of Genetic Counseling, 30,* 574–587.

Betcher, D. K. (2010). Elephant in the Room Project: Improving caring efficacy through effective and compassionate communication with palliative care patients. *Medsurg Nursing, 19,* 101–105.

Bloom, B. S., Englehart, M. D., Furst, E. J., Hill, W. H., & Krathwohl, D. R. (1956). *Taxonomy of educational objectives: Handbook I. Cognitive domain.* David McKay.

Blount, A. J., Taylor, D. D., Lambie, G. W., & Anwell, A. N. (2016). Clinical supervisors' perceptions of wellness: A phenomenological view on supervisee wellness. *The Professional Counselor, 6,* 360–374.

Borders, L. D. (2014). Best practices in clinical supervision: Another step in delineating effective supervision practice. *American Journal of Psychotherapy, 68,* 151–162.

Borders, L. D., Eubanks, S., & Callanan, N. (2006). Supervision of psychosocial skills in genetic counseling. *Journal of Genetic Counseling, 15,* 211–223.

Bosco, A. F. (2000). Caring for the care-giver: The benefit of a peer supervision group. *Journal of Genetic Counseling, 9,* 425–430.

Boysen, G. A., Sampo, B. L., Axtell, E. L., & Kishimoto, A. G. (2022). Disliking students: The experiences and perspectives of college teachers. *College Teaching, 70,* 57–64. doi:10.1080/87567555.2021.1882374

Brainy Quote. (n.d.-a). *Anthony Fauci quotes.* Retrieved April 5, 2021, from https://www.brainyquote.com/quotes/anthony_fauci_652730

Brainy Quote. (n.d.-b). *Edward de Bono quotes.* Retrieved June 22, 2021, from https://www.brainyquote.com/authors/edward-de-bono-quotes

Bubenzer, D., & West, J. (1993). Three supervision modalities for training marital and family counselors. *Counselor Education and Supervision, 33,* 127–138.

Burian, B. K., & O'Connor Slimp, A. (2000). Social dual-role relationships during internship: A decision making model. *Professional Psychology, 31,* 332–338.

Caldwell, S., Wusik, K., He, H., Yager, G., & Atzinger, C. (2018a). Development and validation of the Genetic Counseling Self-Efficacy Scale (GCSES). *Journal of Genetic Counseling, 27,* 1248–1257.

Caldwell, S., Wusik, K., He, H., Yager, G., & Atzinger, C. (2018b). The relationship between the supervisory working alliance and student self-efficacy in genetic counseling training. *Journal of Genetic Counseling, 27,* 1506–1514.

Callanan, N., McCarthy Veach, P., & LeRoy, B. S. (2016). The evolution of clinical supervision in genetic counseling: Theory, research, and practice. *The Clinical Supervisor, 35,* 210–226.

Cambridge Dictionary. (2021). Psychosocial. Retrieved March 17, 2021, from https://dictionary.cambridge.org/dictionary/english/psychosocial

Campinha-Bacote, J. (1994). *The process of cultural competence in health care: A culturally competent model of care.* Transcultural CARE Associates.

Camphina-Bacote, J. (2018). Cultural competemility: A paradigm shift in the cultural competence versus cultural humility debate—Part I. *Online Journal of Issues in Nursing, 24*(1). https://www.doi.org/10.3912/OJIN.Vol24No01PPT20

Carmichael, N., Birnbaum, S., & Redlinger-Grosse, K. (2021). Supporting a sense of inclusion and belonging for genetic counseling students who identify as racial or ethnic minorities.

Journal of Genetic Counseling, 30, 813–827. doi:10.1002/jgc4.1381

Carmichael, N., Redlinger-Grosse, K., & Birnbaum, S. (2020). Conscripted curriculum: The experiences of minority genetic counseling students. *Journal of Genetic Counseling, 29,* 303–314. https://doi.org/10.1002/jgc4.1260

Carmichael, N., Redlinger-Grosse, K., & Birnbaum, S. (2022). Examining clinical training through a bicultural lens: Experiences of genetic counseling students who identify with a racial or ethnic minority group. *Journal of Genetic Counseling, 31*(2), 411–423. doi:10.1002/jgc4.1506

Carraccio, C. L., Benson, B. J., Nixon, L. J., & Derstine, P. L. (2008). From the educational bench to the clinical bedside: translating the Dreyfus developmental model to the learning of clinical skills. *Academic Medicine, 83*(8), 761–767.

Cerney, M. S. (1985). Countertransference revisited. *Journal of Counseling and Development, 63,* 362–364.

Chartered Institute of Personnel and Development. (n.d.). *What is reflective practice?* Retrieved March 14, 2021, from https://beta.cipd uat.co.uk/Images/reflective-practice-guide_tcm18-12524.pdf

Cimino, A. N., Rorke, J., & Adams, H. L. (2013). Supervisors behaving badly: Witnessing ethical dilemmas and what to do about it. *Journal of Social Work Values and Ethics, 10,* 48–57.

Cognology. (n.d.). *49 best quotes on feedback.* Retrieved February 18, 2021, from https://www.cognology.com.au/49-best-quotes-on-feedback

Constantine, M. G. (1997). Facilitating multicultural competency in counseling supervision: Operationalizing a practical framework. In D. B. Pope-Davis & H. L. K. Coleman (Eds.), Multicultural counseling competencies (pp. 310–324). Sage.

Cook, D. A. (1994). Racial identity in supervision. *Counselor Education and Supervision, 34,* 132–141.

Costa, L. (1994). Reducing anxiety in live supervision. *Counselor Education and Supervision, 34,* 30–40.

Cross, T. (1988, Fall). Cultural competence continuum. *Focal Point, 3,* 1–12. https://www.pathwaysrtc.pdx.edu/pdf/fpF88.pdf

Curtis, D. F., Elkins, S. R., Duran, P., & Venta, A. C. (2016). Promoting a climate of reflective practice and clinician self-efficacy in vertical supervision. *Training and Education in Professional Psychology, 10,* 133–140.

Curtis, R. C. (2000). Using goal-setting strategies to enrich the practicum and internship experiences of beginning counseling students. *Journal of Humanistic Counseling, Education and Development, 38*, 194–205.

Danso, R. (2016). Cultural competence and cultural humility: A critical reflection on key cultural diversity concepts. *Journal of Social Work, 18*, 410–430.

Day-Vines, N. L., Ammah, B. B., Steen, S., & Arnold, K. M. (2018). Getting comfortable with discomfort: Preparing counselor trainees to broach racial, ethnic, and cultural factors with clients during counseling. *International Journal for the Advancement of Counselling, 40*, 89–104.

de Leon, A., McCarthy Veach, P., Bro, D., & LeRoy, B. S. (2022). Spanish language concordance in genetic counseling sessions in the United States: Counselor experiences and perceptions of its effects on processes and outcomes. *Journal of Genetic Counseling, 31*, 188–205. https://doi.org/10.1002/jgc4.1472

Dewane, C. J. (2007). Supervisor, beware: Ethical dangers in supervision. *Social Work Today, 7*, 34–40.

Dewey, C., McCarthy Veach, P., LeRoy, B., & Redlinger-Grosse, K. (2022). Experiences of United States genetic counseling supervisors regarding race/ethnicity in supervision: Qualitative investigation. *Journal of Genetic Counseling, 31*(2), 510–522. doi:10.1002/jgc4.1521

Dickerson, J., Vila, P., & Whiticar, R. (2017). The role for peer-assisted ultrasound teaching in medical school. *The Clinical Teacher, 14*, 170–174.

Djurdjinovic, L. (2009). Psychosocial counseling. In W. R. Uhlmann, J. L. Schuette, & B. Yashar (Eds.), *A guide to genetic counseling* (2nd ed., pp. 133–176). Wiley.

Ellis, M. V. (2010). Bridging the science and practice of clinical supervision: Some discoveries, some misconceptions. *The Clinical Supervisor, 29*, 95–116.

Ellis, M. V., Berger, L., Hanus, A. E., Ayala, E. E., Swords, B. A., & Siembor, M. (2013). Inadequate and harmful clinical supervision: Testing a revised framework and assessing occurrence. *The Counseling Psychologist, 42*, 434–472.

English Oxford Living Dictionary. (n.d.). Retrieved September 23, 2019, from https://en.oxforddictionaries.com

Erby, L. A. H., Roter, D. L., & Biesecker, B. B. (2011). Examination of standardized patient performance: Accuracy and consistency of six standardized patients over time. *Patient Education and Counseling, 85,* 194–200.

Ericsson, K. A., & Lehmann, A. C. (1996). Expert and exceptional performance: Evidence of maximal adaptation to task constraints. *Annual Review of Psychology, 47,* 273–305.

Estrada, D., Wiggins Frame, M., & Braun Williams, C. (2004). Cross-cultural supervision: Guiding the conversation toward race and ethnicity. *Journal of Multicultural Counseling and Development, 32,* 307–319.

Eubanks Higgins, S., McCarthy Veach, P., MacFarlane, I. M., Borders, L. D., LeRoy, B. S., & Callanan, N. (2013). Genetic counseling supervisor competencies: Results of a Delphi study. *Journal of Genetic Counseling, 22,* 39–57.

Eurich, T. (2018, January 4). What self-awareness really is and how to cultivate it. *Harvard Business Review.* https://hbr.org/2018/01/what-self-awareness-really-is-and-how-to-cultivate-it

Everyday Power. (n.d.). *Goals quotes: Inspirational sayings on setting goals.* Retrieved February 9, 2021, from https://everydaypower.com/goals-quotes

Falender, C. A., Collins, C. J., & Shafranske, E. P. (2009). "Impairment" and performance issues in clinical supervision: After the 2008 ADA Amendments Act. *Training and Education in Professional Psychology, 3,* 240–249.

Falender, C. A., & Shafranske, E. P. (2021). *Clinical supervision: A competency-based approach* (2nd ed.). American Psychological Association.

Falender, C. A., Shafranske, E. P., & Ofek, A. (2014). Competent clinical supervision: Emerging effective practices. *Counselling Psychology Quarterly, 27,* 393–408.

Fall, M., & Sutton, J. M., Jr. (2004). *Clinical supervision: A handbook for practitioners.* Pearson.

Finley, L. S., McCarthy Veach, P., MacFarlane, I. M., LeRoy, B. S., & Callanan, N. (2016). Perceptions of self-efficacy regarding feedback and goal-setting competencies among genetic counseling clinical supervisors. *Journal of Genetic Counseling, 25,* 344–358.

Fisher-Borne, M., Cain, J. M., & Martin, S. L. (2015). From mastery to accountability: Cultural humility as an alternative to cultural competence. *Social Work Education, 34,* 165–181.

Folkman, S., & Lazarus, R. S. (1985). If it changes it must be a process: Study of emotion and coping during three stages of a college examination. *Journal of Personality and Social Psychology, 48,* 150–170.

Forrest, L., Elman, N., Gizara, S., & Vacha-Haase, T. (1999). Trainee impairment: A review of identification, remediation, dismissal, and legal issues. *The Counseling Psychologist, 27,* 627–686.

French, J. C., Colbert, C. Y., Pien, L. C., Dannefer, E. F., & Taylor, C. A. (2015). Targeted feedback in the milestones era: Utilization of the ask–tell–ask feedback model to promote reflection and self-assessment. *Journal of Surgical Education, 72,* e274–e279.

Friedlander, N. L., Siegel, M., & Brenock, K. (1989). Parallel process in counseling and supervision: A case study. *Journal of Counseling Psychology, 36,* 149–157.

Gallegos, J. (1982). The ethnic competence model for social work education. In B. W. White (Ed.), *Color in a White society* (pp. 1–9). National Association of Social Workers.

Goldsmith, C., Honeywell, C., & Mettler, G. (2011). Peer Observed Interaction and Structured Evaluation (POISE): A Canadian experience with peer supervision for genetic counselors. *Journal of Genetic Counseling, 20,* 204–214.

Goodyear, R. K., Wampold, B. E., Tracey, T. J. G., & Lichtenberg, J. W. (2017). Psychotherapy expertise should mean superior outcomes and demonstrate improvement over time. *The Counseling Psychologist, 45,* 54–65.

Gordon, C., & Luke, M. (2012). Discursive negotiation of face via email: Professional identity development in school counseling supervision. *Linguistics & Education, 23,* 112–122.

Gordon, C., & Luke, M. (2013). Re- and pre-authoring experiences in email supervision: Creating and revising professional meanings in an asynchronous medium. In D. Tannen & A. M. Trester (Eds.), *Discourse 2.0: Language and new media* (pp. 167–181). Georgetown University Press.

Grant, J., Schofield, M. J., & Crawford, S. (2012). Managing difficulties in supervision: Supervisors' perspectives. *Journal of Counseling Psychology, 59,* 528–541.

Gray, L. A., Ladany, N., Walker, J. A., & Ancis, J. R. (2001). Psychotherapy trainees' experience of counterproductive events in supervision. *Journal of Counseling Psychology, 48,* 371.

Grove, M. E., White, S., Fisk, D. G., Rego, S., Dagan-Rosenfeld, O., Kohler, J. N., Reuter, C. M., Bonner, D., Undiagnosed Diseases Network, Wheeler, M. T., Bernstein, J. A., Ormond, K. E., & Hanson-Kahn, A. K. (2019). Developing a genomics rotation: Practical training around variant interpretation for genetic counseling students. *Journal of Genetic Counseling, 28*, 466–476.

Gu, L., McCarthy Veach, P., Eubanks, S., LeRoy, B. S., & Callanan, N. (2011). Boundary issues and multiple relationships in genetic counseling supervision: Supervisor, non-supervisor, and student perspectives. *Journal of Genetic Counseling, 20*, 35–48.

Guy, C. (2016). Genetic counseling milestones: A framework for student competency evaluation. *Journal of Genetic Counseling, 25*, 635–643.

Hart, G., & Nance, D. (2003). Styles of counselor supervision as perceived by supervisors and supervisees. *Counselor Education & Supervision, 43*, 146–158.

Hayden, J., Smiley, R., Alexander, M., Kardong-Edgren, S., & Jeffries, P. (2014). The NCSBN national simulation study: A longitudinal, randomized, controlled study replacing clinical hours with simulation in prelicensure nursing education. *Journal of Nursing Regulation, 5*, S3–S40.

Hays, D. G., & Chang, C. Y. (2003). White privilege, oppression, and racial identity development: Implications for supervision. *Counselor Education & Supervision, 43*, 134–145.

Hays, P. (1996). Addressing the complexities of counseling and gender in counseling. *Journal of Counseling and Development, 74*, 332–338.

Hays, P. (2008). *Addressing cultural complexities in practice: Assessment, diagnosis, and therapy* (2nd ed.). American Psychological Association.

Hendrickson, S. M., McCarthy Veach, P., & LeRoy, B. S. (2002). A qualitative investigation of student and supervisor perceptions of live supervision in genetic counseling. *Journal of Genetic Counseling, 11*, 25–49.

Hess, A. K. (1986). Growth in supervision: Stages of supervisee and supervisor development [Special issue]. *The Clinical Supervisor, 4*(1–2), 51–67.

Hess, A. K. (1987). Psychotherapy supervision: Stages, Buber, and a theory of relationship. *Professional Psychology, 18*, 251–259.

Hill, C. E., Kivlighan, D. M., III, Rousmaniere, T., Kivlighan, D. M., Jr., Gerstenblith, J. A., & Hillman, J. W. (2019). Deliberate practice for the skill of immediacy: A multiple case study of doctoral student therapists and clients. *Psychotherapy, 57*, 587–597.

Hill, C. E., Spiegel, S. B., Hoffman, M. A., Kivlighan, D. M., Jr., & Gelso, C. J. (2017). Therapist expertise in psychotherapy revisited. *The Counseling Psychologist, 45*, 7–53.

Hiller, E., & Rosenfield, J. M. (2000). The experience of leader-led peer supervision: Genetic counselors' perspectives. *Journal of Genetic Counseling, 9*, 399–410.

Hoffman, M. A., Hill, C. E., Holmes, S. E., & Freitas, G. F. (2005). Supervisor perspective on the process and outcome of giving easy, difficult, or no feedback to supervisees. *Journal of Counseling Psychology, 52*, 3–13.

Hofsess, C. D., & Tracey, T. J. G. (2010). Countertransference as a prototype: The development of a measure. *Journal of Counseling Psychology, 57*, 52–67.

Holt, H., Beutler, L. E., Kimpara, S., Macias, S., Haug, N. A., Shiloff, N., Goldblum, P., Sealey Temkin, S., & Stein, M. (2015). Evidence-based supervision: Tracking outcome and teaching principles of change in clinical supervision to bring science to integrative practice. *Psychotherapy, 52*, 185–189.

Holt, R. L., Tofil, N. M., Hurst, C., Youngblood, A. Q., Taylor Peterson, D., Zinkan, J. L., White, M. L., Clemons, J. L., & Robin, N. H. (2013). Utilizing high-fidelity crucial conversation simulation in genetic counseling training. *American Journal of Medical Genetics Part A, 161A*, 1273–1277.

Hou, J. M., & Skovholt, T. M. (2020). Characteristics of highly resilient therapists. *Journal of Counseling Psychology, 67*, 386–400.

Howard, F. (2008). Managing stress or enhancing wellbeing? Positive psychology's contributions to clinical supervision. *Australian Psychologist, 43*, 105–113.

International Nursing Association for Clinical Simulation and Learning Standards Committee. (2016, December). INACSL standards of best practice: Simulation simulation design. *Clinical Simulation in Nursing, 12*(Suppl.), S5–S12. http://dx.doi.org/10.1016/j.ecns.2016.09.005

Jacobs, S. C., Huprichs, S. K., Grus, C. L., Cage, C. A., Elman, N. S., Forrest, L., Schwartz-Mette, R., Shen-Miller, D., Van Sickle, K., & Kaslow, N. J. (2011). Trainees with professional competency problems: Preparing trainers for difficult but necessary conversations. *Training and Education in Professional Psychology, 5,* 175–184.

Janson, G. R. (1998, September). A journey to a theory. *Counseling Today,* 46.

Jungbluth, C., MacFarlane, I. M., McCarthy Veach, P., & LeRoy, B. S. (2011). Why is everyone so anxious? An exploration of stress and anxiety in genetic counseling graduate students. *Journal of Genetic Counseling, 20,* 270–286.

Kagan, N. (1971). *Influencing human interaction.* Instructional Media Center, Michigan State University.

Kagan, N., & Schauble, P. G. (1969). Affect stimulation in interpersonal process recall. *Journal of Counseling Psychology, 16,* 309–313.

Karon, J. (2017). *To be where you are.* Putnam.

Kennedy, A. L. (2000a). Supervision for practicing genetic counselors: An overview of models. *Journal of Genetic Counseling, 9,* 379–390.

Kennedy, A. L. (2000b). A leader-led supervision group as a model for practicing genetic counselors. *Journal of Genetic Counseling, 9,* 391–397.

Keppers, R., McCarthy Veach, P., MacFarlane, I. M., Schema, L., & LeRoy, B. S. (2022). Differences in genetic counseling student responses to intense patient affect: A study of genetic counseling graduate students training in North American programs. *Journal of Genetic Counseling, 31*(2), 398–410. https://doi.org/10.1002/jgc4.1505

Kessler, L. J., LaMarra, D., MacFarlane, I. M., Heller, M., & Valverde, K. D. (2021). Characterizing standardized patients and genetic counseling graduate education. *Journal of Genetic Counseling, 30,* 493–502.

Kessler, S. (1992). Psychological aspects of genetic counseling. VIII. Suffering and countertransference. *Journal of Genetic Counseling, 1,* 303–308.

Kessler, S. (2000). Letter to the editor: Emotional rescue. *Journal of Genetic Counseling, 9,* 275–277.

King, K. (2019). "I want to, but how?" Defining counselor broaching in core tenets and debated components. *Journal of Multicultural Counseling and Development, 49,* 87–100.

Knox, S. (2015). Disclosure—and lack thereof—in individual supervision. *The Clinical Supervisor, 34,* 151–163.

Koehn, P., & Swick, H. (2006). Medical education for a changing world: Moving beyond cultural competence into transnational competence. *Academic Medicine, 81,* 548–556.

Krueger, W. K. (2014). *Windigo Island.* Atria.

Kuo, H. J., Connor, A., Landon, T. J., & Chen, R. K. (2016). Managing anxiety in clinical supervision. *Journal of Rehabilitation, 82,* 18–27.

Ladany, N., Hill, C. E., Corbett, M. M., & Nutt, E. A. (1996). Nature, extent, and importance of what psychotherapy trainees do not disclose to their supervisors. *Journal of Counseling Psychology, 43,* 10–24.

Lamb, D. H., Cochran, D. J., & Jackson, V. R. (1991). Training and organizational issues associated with identifying and responding to intern impairment. *Professional Psychology, 22,* 291–296.

Lanning, W. (1986). Development of the supervisor emphasis rating form. *Counselor Education & Supervision, 25,* 191–196.

Lee, H. K., McCarthy Veach, P., & LeRoy, B. S. (2009). An investigation of relationships among genetic counselors' supervision skills and multicultural counseling competence. *Journal of Genetic Counseling, 18,* 287–299.

Lee, M. J. (2016). On patient safety: When are we too old to operate? *Clinical Orthopaedics and Related Research, 474,* 895–898.

Lee, W., McCarthy Veach, P., MacFarlane, I. M., & LeRoy, B. S. (2014). Who is at risk for compassion fatigue? An investigation of genetic counselor demographics, anxiety, compassion satisfaction, and burnout. *Journal of Genetic Counseling, 24,* 358–370.

Lehrman-Waterman, D., & Ladany, N. (2001). Development and validation of the Evaluation Process Within Supervision Inventory. *Journal of Counseling Psychology, 48,* 168–177.

Leininger, M. (1978). *Transcultural nursing: Concepts, theories, and practices.* Wiley.

Lenz, A. S., & Smith, R. L. (2010). Integrating wellness concepts within a clinical supervision model. *The Clinical Supervisor, 29,* 228–245.

Lewis, K. L., Bohnert, C. A., Gammon, W. L., Holzer, H., Lyman, L., Smith, C., Thompson, T. M., Wallace, A., & Gilva-McConvey, G. (2017). The Association of Standardized Patient Educations (ASPE) standards of best practice (SOBP). *Advances in Simulation, 2,* 1–8.

Lewis, K. L., Erby, L. A. H., Bergner, A. L., Reed, E. K., Johnson, M. R., Adcock, J. Y., & Weaver, M. A. (2017). The dynamics of a genetic counseling peer supervision. *Journal of Genetic Counseling, 26,* 532–540.

Liddle, B. J. (1986). Resistance in supervision: A response to perceived threat. *Counselor Education and Supervision, 26,* 117–127.

Lindh, H., McCarthy Veach, P., Cikanek, K., & LeRoy, B. S. (2003). A survey of clinical supervision in genetic counseling. *Journal of Genetic Counseling, 12,* 23–41.

Loganbill, C., Hardy, E., & Delworth, U. (1982). Supervision: A conceptual model. *The Counseling Psychologist, 10,* 3–42.

Lu, C., & Wan, C. (2018). Cultural self-awareness as awareness of culture's influence on the self: Implications for cultural identification and well being. *Personality and Social Psychology Bulletin, 44,* 823–837.

Luke, M., & Gordon, C. (2011). A discourse analysis of school counseling supervisory email. *Counselor Education and Supervision, 50,* 274–291.

Luke, M., & Gordon, C. (2016). Clinical supervision via e-mail. In T. Rousmaniere & E. Renfro-Michel (Eds.), *Using technology to enhance clinical supervision* (pp. 117–134). American Counseling Association.

MacFarlane, I. M. (2013). *Anxiety's effect on the experience of supervision of genetic counseling students.* University of Minnesota Digital Conservancy. https://conservancy.umn.edu/bitstream/handle/11299/167261

MacFarlane, I. M., McCarthy Veach, P., Grier, J. E., Meister, D. J., & LeRoy, B. S. (2016). Effects of anxiety on novice genetic counseling students' experience of supervision. *Journal of Genetic Counseling, 25,* 742–766.

MacLeod, L. (2012). Making SMART goals smarter. *Physician Executive, 38*(2), 68.

Mager, R. F. (1997). *Preparing instructional objectives* (3rd ed.). CEP Press.

Magnusson, S., Wilcoxen, S. A., & Norem, K. (2000). A profile of lousy supervision: Experienced counselors' perspectives. *Counselor Education and Supervision, 39,* 189–202.

Martin, P., Copley, J., & Tyacki, Z. (2014). Twelve tips for effective clinical supervision based on a narrative literature review and expert opinion. *Medical Teacher, 36,* 201–207.

Martin, P., Kumar, S., & Lizarondo, L. (2017). Effective use of technology in clinical supervision. *Internet Interventions, 8,* 35–39.

Masunga, A., Wusik, K., He, H., Yager, G., & Atzinger, C. (2014). Barriers impacting the utilization of supervision techniques in genetic counseling. *Journal of Genetic Counseling, 23*, 992–1001.

Mateo, C. M., & Williams, D. R. (2020). More than words: A vision to address bias and reduce discrimination in the health professions learning environment. *Academic Medicine, 95*, S169–S177.

McCarthy Veach, P. (2001). Conflict and counterproductivity in supervision: When relationships are less than ideal: Comment on Nelson and Friedlander (2001) and Gray et al. (2001). *Journal of Counseling Psychology, 48*, 396–400.

McCarthy Veach, P. (2021). Goal setting in genetic counseling supervision: Basic concepts and skills module. In *Supervision of genetic counseling students: How and why*. Association of Genetic Counseling Program Directors. http://media.mycrowdwisdom.com.s3.amazon aws.com/nsgc/Supervision%20Modules/scormcontent/index.html

McCarthy Veach, P., Bartels, D. M., & LeRoy, B. S. (2007). Coming full circle: A Reciprocal-Engagement Model of genetic counseling practice. *Journal of Genetic Counseling, 16*, 713–728.

McCarthy Veach, P., & LeRoy, B. S. (2009). Student supervision: Strategies for providing direction, guidance, and support. In W. R. Uhlmann, J. L. Schuette, & B. Yashar (Eds.), *A guide to genetic counseling* (2nd ed., pp. 401–434). Wiley.

McCarthy Veach, P., LeRoy, B. S., & Callanan, N. P. (2018). *Facilitating the genetic counseling process: Practice-based skills* (2nd ed.). Springer.

McCarthy Veach, P., Willaert, R., & LeRoy, B. S. (2009). *Giving and receiving feedback in supervision: A DVD workbook*. University of Minnesota, Minneapolis, MN.

McCarthy Veach, P., Yoon, E., Miranda, C., Macfarlane, I., Ergun, D., & Tuicomepee, A. (2012). Clinical supervisor value conflicts: Low frequency, but high impact events. *The Clinical Supervisor, 31*, 203–227.

McIntosh, N., Dircks, A., Fitzpatrick, J., & Shuman, C. (2006). Games in clinical genetic counseling supervision. *Journal of Genetic Counseling, 15*, 225–244.

Meghani, D. T., & Ferm, B. R. (2021). Development of a standardized patient evaluation exam: An innovative model for health service psychology programs. *Training and Education in Professional Psychology, 15*, 37–44.

Mehr, K. E., Ladany, N., & Caskie, G. I. L. (2010). Trainee nondisclo-sure in supervision: What are they not telling you? *Counselling and Psychotherapy Research, 10,* 103–113.

Merriam-Webster. (n.d.-a). Resilience. In *Merriam-Webster.com dictionary.* Retrieved April 14, 2021, from https://www.merriam-webster.com/dictionary/resilience

Merriam-Webster. (n.d.-b). Stress. In *Merriam-Webster.com dictionary.* Retrieved April 14, 2021, from https://www.merriam-webster.com/dictionary/stress

Middleton, A., Wiles, V., Kershaw, A., Everest, S., Downing, S., Burton, H., Robathan, S., & Landy, A. (2007). Reflections on the experience of counseling supervision by a team of genetic counselors from the UK. *Journal of Genetic Counseling, 16,* 143–155.

Miller, S., Nunnally, E., & Wackman, D. (1975). *Alive and aware.* Interpersonal Communications.

Minnes, P. M. (1989). Ethical issues in supervision. *Canadian Psychology, 28,* 285–290.

Miranda, C., McCarthy Veach, P., Martyr, M., & LeRoy, B. S. (2016). Portrait of the master genetic counselor: A qualitative inves-tigation of expertise in genetic counseling. *Journal of Genetic Counseling, 25,* 767–785.

Moffett, L. (2009). Directed self-reflection protocols in supervision. *Training and Education in Professional Psychology, 3,* 78–83.

Moncho, C. (2013, August 10). Structuring supervision. *The Social Work Practitioner.* Retrieved January 21, 2021, from https://thesocialworkpractitioner.com/2013/08/10/structuring-supervision

Myers, J. E., Sweeney, T. J., & Witmer, J. M. (2000). The wheel of wellness counseling for wellness: A holistic model for treatment planning. *Journal of Counseling and Development, 78,* 251–266.

National Society of Genetic Counselors. (2018). National Society of Genetic Counselors code of ethics. *Journal of Genetic Counseling, 27,* 6–8.

National Society of Genetic Counselors. (2020). *Professional Status Survey 2020: Work environment.* NSGC Executive Office.

National Society of Genetic Counselors. (2021). *Promoting cultural competency within NSGC.* https://www.nsgc.org/page/culturalcompetency

Nelson, M. L., & Friedlander, M. L. (2001). A close look at conflictual supervisory relationships: The trainee's perspective. *Journal of Counseling Psychology, 48,* 384–395.

Neville, H., Spanierman, L., & Doan, B. T. (2006). Exploring the association between color-blind racial ideology and multicultural counseling competencies. *Cultural Diversity and Ethnic Minority Psychology, 12*(2), 275.

Norman, R. L. (2015). The intentional use of the parallel process during cross-cultural counseling supervision. *VISTAS Online, 5*(55), 1–12.

Orchowski, L., Evangelista, N. M., & Probst, D. R. (2010). Enhancing supervisee reflectivity in clinical supervision: A case study illustration. *Psychotherapy Theory, Research, Practice, Training, 47,* 51–67.

Overholser, J. C. (2004). The four pillars of psychotherapy supervision. *The Clinical Supervisor, 23,* 1–13.

Overholser, J. C., & Fine, M. A. (1990). Defining the boundaries of professional competence: Managing subtle cases of clinical incompetence. *Professional Psychology, 21,* 462–469.

Pangaro, L. (1999). A new vocabulary and other innovations for improving descriptive in-training evaluations. *Academic Medicine, 74,* 1203–1207.

Pangaro, L., & Cate, O. T. (2013). Frameworks for learner assessment in medicine: AMEE Guide No. 78. *Medical Teacher, 35,* e1197–e1210.

Papps, E., & Ramsden, I. (1996). Cultural safety in nursing: The New Zealand experience. *International Journal of Quality in Health Care, 8,* 491–497.

Paramasivan, A., & Khoo, D. (2019). Standardized patients versus peer role play-exploring the experience, efficacy, and cost-effectiveness in residency training module for breaking bad news. *Journal of Surgical Education, 77,* 479–484.

Pearson, Q. M. (2001). A case in clinical supervision: A framework for putting theory into practice. *Journal of Mental Health Counseling, 23,* 174–183.

Penny, L. (2013). *The beautiful music.* Minotaur.

Peters, H. C. (2017). Multicultural supervision: An intersectional lens for clinical supervision. *International Journal of the Advancement of Counselling, 39,* 176–187.

Polanski, P. (2000, Winter). Training supervisors at the master's level: Developmental considerations. *ACES Spectrum Newsletter*, 3–5.

Pope, K. S., & Vasquez, M. J. T. (2010). *Ethics in psychotherapy and counseling: A practical guide*. Wiley

Purnell, L. (2002). The Purnell Model for Cultural Competence. *Journal of Transcultural Nursing, 13*(3), 193–196.

Purnell, L., & Paulanka, B. (1998). *Transcultural health care: A culturally competent approach*. Davis.

Ramos-Sánchez, L., Esnil, E., Goodwin, A., Riggs, S., Touster, L. O., Wright, L. K., Ratanasiripong, P., & Rodolfa, E. (2002). Negative supervisory events: Effects on supervision and supervisory alliance. *Professional Psychology, 33*, 197–202.

Redlinger-Grosse, K. (2020). Countertransference: Making the unconscious conscious. In B. S. LeRoy, P. McCarthy Veach, & N. P. Callanan (Eds.), *Genetic counseling practice: Advanced concepts and skills* (2nd ed., pp. 153–176). Wiley.

Redlinger-Grosse, K., Anderson, K., Birkeland, L., Zaleski, C., & Reiser, C. (2021). 6 feet apart but working together. *Journal of Genetic Counseling, 30*(4), 1069–1073. https://doi.org/10.1002/jgc4.1408

Redlinger-Grosse, K., McCarthy Veach, P., LeRoy, B. S., & Zierhut, H. (2017). Elaboration of the Reciprocal-Engagement Model of genetic counseling practice: A qualitative investigation of goals and strategies. *Journal of Genetic Counseling, 26*, 1372–1387.

Reeder, R., McCarthy Veach, P., MacFarlane, I. M., & LeRoy, B. S. (2017). Characterizing clinical genetic counselors' countertransference experiences: An exploratory study. *Journal of Genetic Counseling, 26*, 934–947.

Reiser, C. (2019). Genetic counseling clinical supervision: A call to action. *Journal of Genetic Counseling, 28*, 727–729.

Reiser, C. A. (2021). "Oh the places you'll go!" The genetic counselor professional development journey. In B. S. LeRoy, P. McCarthy Veach, & N. P. Callanan (Eds.), *Genetic counseling practice: Advanced concepts and skills* (2nd ed., pp. 341–360). Wiley.

Resta, R. (2002). Commentary on the inner world of the genetic counselor: The unexamined counseling life. *Journal of Genetic Counseling, 11*, 19–24.

Roche, M. I., & Greb, A. (2016). It's time to ramp up genetic counseling training. *Genetics in Medicine, 18*, 768–769.

Rodenhauser, P. (1994). Toward a multidimensional model for psycho-therapy supervision based on developmental stages. *Journal of Psychotherapy Practice and Research, 3,* 1–15.

Rodenhauser, P. (1997). Psychotherapy supervision: Prerequisites and problems in the process. In C. E. Watkins (Ed.), *Handbook of psychotherapy supervision* (pp. 527–548). Wiley.

Ruiz-Moral, R., Perula de Torres, L., Monge, D., Garcia Leonardo, C., & Caballero, F. (2017). Teaching medical students to express empathy by exploring patient emotions and experiences in standardized medical encounters. *Patient Education and Counseling, 100,* 1694–1700.

Russell, C. S., DuPree, W. J., Beggs, M. A., Peterson, C. M., & Anderson, M. P. (2007). Responding to remediation and gate-keeping challenges in supervision. *Journal of Marital and Family Therapy, 33,* 227–244.

Sahebi, B. (2020). Clinical supervision of couple and family therapy during COVID-19. *Family Process, 59,* 989–996.

Santana, M. C., & Fouad, N. A. (2017). Development and validation of a self-care behavior inventory. *Training and Education in Professional Psychology, 11,* 140–145.

Schon, D. A. (1991). *The reflective practitioner* (2nd ed.). Jossey-Bass.

Schoonveld, K. S., McCarthy Veach, P., & LeRoy, B. S. (2007). What is it like to be in the minority? Ethnic and gender diversity in the genetic counseling profession. *Journal of Genetic Counseling, 16,* 53–70.

Schultz, K., Singer, A., & Oadansan, I. (2021). Seven topics for clinical supervision in the time of COVID 19. *Canadian Medical Education Journal, 12,* e81–e84.

Scraper, R. L. (2000). The art and science of maieutic questioning within the Socratic method. *International Forum for Logotherapy, 23,* 14–16.

Secton, A., Hodgkin, L., Bogwitz, M., Bylstra, Y., Mann, K., Taylor, J., Hodgson, J., Sahhar, M., & Kentwell, M. (2013). A model for peer experiential and reciprocal supervision (PEERS) for genetic counselors: Development and preliminary evaluation within clinical practice. *Journal of Genetic Counseling, 22,* 175–187.

Selman, L. E., Brighton, L. J., Hawkins, A., McDonald, C., O'Brien, S., Robinson, V., Khan, S. A., George, R., Ramsenthaler, C., Higginson, I. J., & Koffman, J. (2017). The effect of communication skills training for generalist palliative care providers on patient-reported outcomes and clinician behaviors: A systematic review and meta-analysis. *Journal of Pain and Symptom Management, 54*, 404–416.

Sevenhuysen, S., Farlie, M. K., Keating, J. L., Haines, T. P., & Molloy, E. (2015). Physiotherapy students and clinical educators perceive several ways in which incorporating peer-assisted learning could improve clinical placements: A qualitative study. *Journal of Physiotherapy, 61*, 87–92.

Sevenhuysen, S., Skinner, E. H., Farlie, M. K., Raitman, L., Nickson, W., Keating, J. L., & Haines, T. P. (2014). Educators and students prefer traditional clinical education to a peer-assisted learning model, despite similar student performance outcomes: A randomised trial. *Journal of Physiotherapy, 60*, 209–216.

Shugar, A. (2017). Teaching genetic counseling skills: Incorporating a genetic counseling adaptation continuum model to address psychosocial complexity. *Journal of Genetic Counseling, 26*, 215–223.

Shulman, L. (2006). The clinical supervisor–practitioner working alliance. *The Clinical Supervisor, 24*, 23–47.

Siskind, C. E., & Atzinger, C. L. (2019). Supervision in genetic counselor training in North America: A systematic review. *Journal of Genetic Counseling, 28*, 1069–1086.

Sitaula, A., McCarthy Veach, P., MacFarlane, I. M., Lee, W., & Redlinger-Grosse, K. (2019 November 5–8). An investigation of genetic counselors' responses to prenatal patient religious/spiritual statements [Paper presentation]. National Society of Genetic Counselors Annual Education Meeting, Salt Lake City, UT.

Slater, R., McCarthy Veach, P., & Li, Z. (2012). Recognizing and managing countertransference in the college classroom: An exploration of expert teachers' experiences. *Innovative Higher Education, 38*, 3–17.

Smith, K. L. (2009). *A brief summary of supervision models.* Retrieved May 31, 2021, from https://www.gallaudet.edu/documents/Dep artment-of-Counseling/COU_SupervisionModels_Rev.pdf

Sotto-Santiago, S., Mac, J., Duncan, F., & Smith, J. (2020). I didn't know what to say": Responding to racism, discrimination, and microaggressions with the OWTFD approach. *MedEdPORTAL, 16*, 10971.

Stake, R. (1977). Formative and summative evaluation. In D. Hamilton, D. Jenkins, C. King, B. MacDonald, & M. Parlett (Eds.), Beyond the *numbers game* (pp. 156–169). Macmillan.

Stoltenberg, C. D., & McNeill, B. W. (2011). *IDM supervision: An integrative developmental model for supervising counselors & therapists.* Routledge.

Stoltenberg, C. D., McNeill, B. W., & Delworth, U. (1998). *IDM: An integrated developmental model for supervising counselors and therapists.* Jossey-Bass.

Students, C., & Pearson, Q. M. (2004). Getting the most out of clinical supervision: Strategies for mental health. *Journal of Mental Health Counseling, 26,* 361–373.

Sue, D. W. (2001). Multidimensional facets of cultural competence. *The Counseling Psychologist, 29*(6), 790–821. https://doi.org/10.1177%2F0011000001296002

Sue, D. W. (2010). *Microaggressions in everyday life: Race, gender, and sexual orientation.* Wiley.

Sue, D. W., Bernier, J. B., Durran, M., Feinberg, L., Pedersen, P., Smith, E., & Vasquez-Nuttall, E. (1982). Position paper: Cross-cultural counseling competencies. *The Counseling Psychologist, 10,* 45–52.

Sue, S., Fujino, D. C., Hu, L. T., Takeuchi, D. T., & Zane, N. W. (1991). Community mental health services for ethnic minority groups: A test of the cultural responsiveness hypothesis. *Journal of Consulting and Clinical Psychology, 59,* 533–540.

Suguitan, M. D., Redlinger-Grosse, K., McCarthy Veach, P., & LeRoy, B. S. (2019). Genetic counseling supervisor strategies: An elaboration of the Reciprocal-Engagement Model of Supervision. *Journal of Genetic Counseling, 28,* 602–615.

Sutton, J. (2020). *Socratic questioning in psychology: Examples and techniques.* Retrieved March 13, 2021, from https://positivepsychology.com/socratic-questioning

Tai, J. H. M., Canny, B. J., Haines, T. P., & Molloy, E. K. (2016). The role of peer-assisted learning in building evaluative judgement: Opportunities in clinical medical educations. *Advances in Health Sciences Education, 21,* 659–676.

Talusan, L. (2021, April). *Action planning for cultural change in genetic counseling.* Minnesota Genetic Counseling Association Semi-Annual Education Conference; conference conducted remotely due to COVID-19.

Tervalon, M., & Murray-Garcia, J. (1998). Cultural humility versus cultural competence: A critical distinction in defining physician training outcomes in multicultural education. *Journal of Health Care for the Poor and Underserved, 9,* 117–125.

Tomlinson, C. A. (2012, November 1). *One to grow on/the evaluation of my dreams*. Association for Supervision and Curriculum Development. Retrieved October 10, 2021, from https://www.ascd.org/el/articles/the-evaluation-of-my-dreams

Townend, M. (2005). Interprofessional supervision from perspectives of both mental health nurses and other professionals in the field of cognitive behavioral psychotherapy. *Journal of Psychiatry and Mental Health Nursing, 12*, 582–588.

Udipi, S., McCarthy Veach, P., Kao, J., & LeRoy, B. S. (2008). The psychic costs of empathic engagement: Personal and demographic predictors of genetic counselor compassion fatigue. *Journal of Genetic Counseling, 17*, 459–471.

Uhlmann, W. R. (2009). Thinking it all through: Case preparation and management. In W. R. Uhlmann, J. L. Schuette, & B. M. Yashar (Eds.), *A guide to genetic counseling* (pp. 93–132). Wiley-Blackwell.

Veilleux, J. C., January, A. M., Vanderveen, J. W., Felice Reddy, L., & Klonoff, E. A. (2012). Differentiating amongst characteristics associated with problems of professional competence: Perceptions of graduate student peers. *Training and Education in Professional Psychology, 6*, 113–121.

Venart, E., Vassos, S., &, Pitcher-Heft, H. (2007). What individual counselors can do to sustain wellness. *Journal of Humanistic Counseling, Education and Development, 46*, 50–65.

Venne, V. L., & Coleman, D. (2010). Training the millennial learner through experiential evolutionary scaffolding: Implications for clinical supervision in graduate education programs. *Journal of Genetic Counseling, 19*, 554–569.

Watkins, C. E., Jr. (1985). Countertransference: Its impact on the counseling situation. *Journal of Counseling and Development, 63*, 356–359.

Watkins, C. E., Jr. (1993). Development of the psychotherapy supervisor: Concepts, assumptions, and hypotheses of the supervisor complexity model. *American Journal of Psychotherapy, 47*, 58–74.

Watkins, C. E., Jr. (1995). Psychotherapy supervisor development: On musings, models, and metaphor. *Journal of Psychotherapy Practice & Research, 4*, 150–158.

Watkins. C. E., Jr. (1997). The ineffective psychotherapy supervisor: Some reflections about bad behaviors. poor process. and offensive outcomes. *The Clinical Supervisor, 16*, 163–180.

Watkins, C. E., Jr. (2012). Development of the psychotherapy supervisor: Review of and reflections on 30 years of theory and research. *American Journal of Psychotherapy, 66,* 45–83.

Watkins, C. E., Jr., Schneider, L. J., Haynes, J., & Nieberding, R. (1995). Measuring psychotherapy supervisor development: An initial effort at scale development and validation. *The Clinical Supervisor, 13,* 77–90.

Weil, J. (2000). Introduction. *Journal of Genetic Counseling, 9,* 375–378.

Weil, J. (2010). Countertransference: Making the unconscious conscious. In B. S. LeRoy, P. McCarthy Veach, & D. M. Bartels (Eds.), *Genetic counseling practice: Advanced concepts and skills* (pp. 175–200). Wiley-Blackwell.

Wells, D., McCarthy Veach, P., Martyr, M., & LeRoy, B. S. (2016). Development, experience, and expression of meaning in genetic counselors' lives: A qualitative investigation. *Journal of Genetic Counseling, 25,* 799–817.

Werner-Lin, A., McCoyd, J. L., & Bernhardt, B. A. (2016). Balancing genetics (science) and counseling (art) in prenatal chromosomal microarray testing. *Journal of Genetic Counseling, 25*(5), 855–867.

Wherley, C., McCarthy Veach, P., Martyr, M., & LeRoy, B. S. (2015). Form follows function: A model for clinical supervision practice in genetic counseling. *Journal of Genetic Counseling, 24,* 702–716.

Winspear, J. (2009). *Among the mad.* Holt.

Winspear, J. (2010). *The mapping of love and death.* HarperCollins.

Wong, L. C. J., Wong, P. T. P., & Ishiyama, F. I. (2013). What helps and what hinders in cross-cultural clinical supervision: A critical incident study. *The Counseling Psychologist, 41,* 66–85. doi:10.1177/0011000012442652

Worthington, R. L., Andreas Tan, J., & Poulin, K. (2002). Ethically questionable behaviors among supervisees: An exploratory investigation. *Ethics and Behavior, 12,* 323–351.

Yager, G. G., Wilson, F. R., Brewer, D., & Kinnetz, P. (1989). *The development and validation of an instrument to measure counseling supervisor focus and style* [Paper presentation]. Annual Meeting of the American Education Research Association, San Francisco. Unpublished instrument.

Yancu, C., & Farmer, D. (2017). Product or process: Cultural competence or cultural humility? *Palliative Medicine and Hospice Care Open Journal, 3*(1), e1–e4. doi:10.17140/PMHCOJ-3-e005

Zahm, K., McCarthy Veach, P., & LeRoy B.S. (2008). An investigation of genetic counselor experiences in peer group supervision. *Journal of Genetic Counseling, 17*, 220–233.

Zahm, K. W., McCarthy Veach, P., Martyr, M., & LeRoy, B. S. (2016). From graduate to seasoned practitioner: A qualitative investigation of genetic counselor professional development. *Journal of Genetic Counseling, 25*, 818–834.

Index

For the benefit of digital users, indexed terms that span two pages (e.g., 52–53) may, on occasion, appear on only one of those pages.

Tables, figures, and boxes are indicated by *t*, *f*, and *b* following the page number

evaluation (*cont.*)
  strategies to promote
    evaluation processes,
    217–19 (*see also* Genetic
    Counseling Self-Efficacy
    Scale)
  summative evaluation, 207
  supervisor competencies, 29–
    30, 221*b*
evocative approaches, 44–45,
  46, 49, 131, 184, 187–88,
  191–92, 193, 229, 238–
  39, 266–67, 349, 377–78,
  381 (*see also* ask-tell-ask-
  model; evocative teaching
  supervisory style; open-
  faced sandwich feedback)

feedback. *See also* evaluation
  evaluation of supervisor skills,
    197–98, 230
  functions, 8, 179–80
  helpful characteristics of,
    183–84
  strategies, 105–6, 184–97 (*see
    also* difficult conversations)
  ask-tell-ask-model, 191–92
  open-faced sandwich, 191
  supervisor competencies, 30,
    32, 35
  types and approaches, 180–82
  corrective, 180*b*, 181–82
  distal, 186–87
  evocative, 187–88 (*see also*
    directive vs. evocative
    teaching supervisory
    style; evocative
    approaches)
  immediate, 186–87
  positive, 180–81

Genetic Counseling Self-Efficacy
  Scale, 215, 223–26
goals
  determining goal content,
    160–61 (*see also* practice-
    based competencies;
    supervision theoretical
    model)
  definition and functions of,
    157–58
  types of performance goals, 158
  viable goal characteristics,
    159, 159*b*
goal accomplishment strategies,
  170–72. *See also*
    formative evaluation;
    summative evaluation
goal setting
  evaluation of supervisor goal
    setting skills, 169–70, 173
  pitfalls, 167–70
  ego-versus task orientation,
    168–69
  implicit expectations,
    167–68
  student developmental
    level, 137*t*
  processes, 159–63
  strategies, 163–70, 262
  supervisor competencies,
    28–29

independent counseling, 148–52
  assessing student readiness
    for, 148–50, 149*b*
  preparing students for,
    150–51
  Reciprocal Engagement Model
    of Supervision outcome
    goal, 6–7